The RAND/UCLA Appropriateness Method User's Manual

Kathryn Fitch
Steven J. Bernstein
María Dolores Aguilar
Bernard Burnand
Juan Ramón LaCalle
Pablo Lázaro
Mirjam van het Loo
Joseph McDonnell
John Paul Vader
James P. Kahan

D1310352

Prepared for Directorate General XII,
European Commission

RAND *Europe*   RAND *Health*

The research described in this report was prepared for Directorate General XII, European Commission.

Library of Congress Cataloging-in-Publication Data

The Rand/UCLA appropriateness method user's manual / Kathryn Fitch ... [et al.].
    p. cm.
    "MR-1269-DG-XII/RE."
    Includes bibliographical references.
    ISBN 0-8330-2918-5
    1. Medical care—Decision making. 2. Medical care—Utilization review. 3. Clinical indications. 4. Delphi method. I. Fitch, Kathryn.

R723.5 .R36 2000
362.1—dc21

                                                                    00-045830

Published 2001 by RAND
1700 Main Street, P.O. Box 2138, Santa Monica, CA 90407-2138
1200 South Hayes Street, Arlington, VA 22202-5050
RAND URL: http://www.rand.org/
To order RAND documents or to obtain additional information, contact Distribution Services: Telephone: (310) 451-7002; Fax: (310) 451-6915; Internet: order@rand.org

PREFACE

The concepts of appropriate and necessary care are fundamental to the creation of an efficient and equitable health-care delivery system. Evidence of inappropriate overuse and underuse of procedures has been documented even in health systems characterised by the absence of global budgets, capitation, utilisation review or the pressure of requiring a second opinion. Health systems should function in such a way that inappropriate care is progressively reduced, while appropriate and especially necessary care are maintained or increased. The ability to determine and identify which care is overused and which is underused is essential to this functioning. To this end, the "RAND/UCLA Appropriateness Method" (here given the acronym RAM) was developed by RAND and UCLA in the 1980s. It has been further developed and refined in North America and, increasingly, in Europe.

This manual presents step-by-step guidelines for conceptualising, designing, and carrying out a study of the appropriateness of medical or surgical procedures (for either diagnosis or treatment) using the RAM. The manual distills the experience of many researchers in North America and Europe, and presents current (as of the year 2000) thinking on the subject. Although the manual is self-contained and as complete as we could make it, the authors do not recommend that someone unfamiliar with the RAM independently conduct an appropriateness study; instead, we strongly advocate a strategy of "seeing one" before "doing one." To this end, the authors of this manual, as well as their collaborators, stand ready to assist potential users of the method. Interested parties should contact one of the authors of this manual (see Annex I for addresses) or, more generally, RAND Health in Santa Monica, California, USA or RAND Europe in Leiden, the Netherlands.

The writing and editing of this manual was carried out as part of the Concerted Action "A method to integrate scientific and clinical knowledge to achieve the appropriate utilisation of major medical and surgical procedures," financed by Directorate General XII of the European Commission under the BIOMED II programme (contract no. BMH4-CT96-0212), during the period 1996-1999.

RAND Health is the health policy unit of RAND. For further information about RAND Health, contact its director, Robert H. Brook.

RAND Europe is the European operating unit of RAND. For further information about RAND Europe, contact its President, David C. Gompert.

Robert H. Brook, MD, ScD
RAND Health
1700 Main Street
P.O. Box 2138
Santa Monica, CA 90407-2138
USA
telephone: +1-310-393-0411
telefax: +1-310-393-4818
e-mail: Robert_Brook@rand.org

David C. Gompert
RAND Europe
Newtonweg 1
2333 CP Leiden
THE NETHERLANDS
telephone: +31-71-524-5151
telefax: +31-71-524-5191
e-mail: info@randeurope.org

CONTENTS

CHAPTER 10

APPLYING APPROPRIATENESS CRITERIA RETROSPECTIVELY TO MEASURE OVERUSE

CHAPTER 11

FIGURES

TABLES

ACKNOWLEDGEMENTS

The RAND/UCLA Appropriateness Method was originally developed at RAND and the UCLA School of Medicine. The authors wish to gratefully acknowledge the creativity of Robert H. Brook in identifying the need to measure the appropriateness and necessity of health care in order to improve its effectiveness, and the pioneering work of Robert H. Brook, Mark Chassin, Arlene Fink, Katherine Kahn, Jackie Kosecoff, Ed Park and David Solomon in developing the RAND/UCLA Appropriateness Method. Our understanding of the method was greatly enhanced by working with many fellow health service researchers, most notably Bobby DuBois, Lucian Leape, Paul Shekelle and Connie Winslow.

Some of the material in this manual has been previously published in RAND documents.

The Concerted Action team (see Annex I for a list of members) encouraged and supported the preparation of this manual. Earlier drafts of the document were read by Ineke van Beusekom, Eduardo Briones, Robert H. Brook, Ignacio Marín León, Herman Stoevelaar and Ernesto Villar; we thank them for their constructive criticism and helpful suggestions.

CHAPTER 1. INTRODUCTION

Background

The RAND/UCLA Appropriateness Method (RAM) was developed in the mid 1980s, as part of the RAND Corporation/University of California Los Angeles (UCLA) Health Services Utilisation Study, primarily as an instrument to enable the measurement of the overuse and underuse of medical and surgical procedures. In the RAM, the concept of appropriateness refers to the relative weight of the benefits and harms of a medical or surgical intervention. An appropriate procedure is one in which "the expected health benefit (e.g., increased life expectancy, relief of pain, reduction in anxiety, improved functional capacity) exceeds the expected negative consequences (e.g., mortality, morbidity, anxiety, pain, time lost from work) by a sufficiently wide margin that the procedure is worth doing, exclusive of cost" (Brook et al., 1986; Park et al., 1986). Robert H. Brook, who identified the need for a tool to measure the appropriateness of care, explained that "it was motivated by the concern that the increasing complexity of medical care was resulting in some patients not undergoing procedures that they needed, and others undergoing procedures that they did not need" (Brook, 1994).

The rationale behind the method is that randomised clinical trials—the "gold standard" for evidence-based medicine—often are either not available or cannot provide evidence at a level of detail sufficient to apply to the wide range of patients seen in everyday clinical practice. Although robust scientific evidence about the benefits of many procedures is lacking, physicians must nonetheless make decisions every day about when to apply them. Consequently, it was believed a method was needed that would combine the best available scientific evidence with the collective judgement of experts to yield a statement regarding the appropriateness of performing a procedure at the level of patient-specific symptoms, medical history and test results.

The appropriateness criteria developed in early RAND studies were used as a tool to measure performance retrospectively: the criteria were applied to representative samples of patients who had received the procedure to determine the proportion of procedures done for inappropriate reasons, that is, to measure overuse. Appropriateness criteria have also come to be used prospectively, as the basis for developing different types of clinical decision aids.

Many procedures have been the subject of appropriateness studies in the United States, among them, coronary angiography, coronary artery bypass graft surgery, percutaneous transluminal coronary angioplasty, carotid endarterectomy, abdominal aortic aneurysm surgery, diagnostic upper gastrointestinal endoscopy, cataract surgery, colonoscopy, cholecystectomy, hysterectomy, tympanostomy and spinal manipulation for lower back pain. The method has since been applied to some of these as well as other conditions and procedures—benign prostatic hyperplasia, laminectomy, breast cancer and total hip replacement—in a wide variety of countries, including Canada, Israel, Italy, The Netherlands, Spain, Sweden, Switzerland, and the United Kingdom. Use continues to expand to other countries, particularly in Western Europe (Kahan and van het Loo, 1999).

An important finding of the early RAND studies was that the differences in the volume of procedures across geographical areas were generally not related with levels of appropriateness (Chassin et al., 1987). A large body of research had documented major variations in the use of procedures among and within geographic regions, and the RAND investigators hypothesised that higher rates of inappropriate use in high-volume areas might explain some of these differences. Surprisingly, it was found that the proportion of inappropriate procedures was not associated with the number of procedures performed. This finding led to the suggestion that both underuse and overuse of procedures might be occurring simultaneously in the same area. In testimony before a US Senate Committee in March 1999, Brook (1999) cited the results of a study in the United Kingdom, where physicians perform only 1/7th the number of cardiac procedures as in the United States and patients are often put on long waiting lists to receive coronary revascularization. The study showed "gross underuse of procedures for people who needed them and gross overuse for people who didn't need them."

To measure underuse, the RAND/UCLA method was expanded to measure the *necessity* of clinical procedures (Kahan et al., 1994a). Necessity is a more stringent criterion than appropriateness and refers to procedures that *must* be offered to patients fitting a particular clinical description. Necessity criteria have been developed for a number of procedures (coronary angiography, coronary revascularization) to measure underuse or "unmet need." Necessity is more difficult to measure than appropriateness, however, because it involves identifying a group of patients who *might* have benefited from the procedure, but did not receive it.

Purpose of this Manual

The purpose of this manual is to explain what the appropriateness method is and how it works. Experience with the RAM is now broad enough, we believe, that prospective new users might benefit from the experiences of those who have been through the process. While not a "cookbook," it is hoped that the explanations and examples included in the manual will serve as a guide to those who are considering applying this method, and will help them avoid some of the problems and pitfalls encountered in previous projects.

Readers of this manual may also want to refer to the annotated bibliography of materials related to the RAM (Van het Loo and Kahan, 1999). This document is a cross-referenced guide to a wide variety of published papers as well as documents from the "grey literature" that refer to the appropriateness method and its applications. Abstracts are included for all documents where they are available. The annotated bibliography is organised into five main categories: Descriptions of the RAND/UCLA Appropriateness Methodology, RAM Outcomes, Within-Panel Comparisons, Multiple-Panel Comparisons, and Non-RAM Studies related to Appropriateness. It provides a valuable resource to persons interested in a more comprehensive study of the appropriateness method.

An Overview of the Method

The basic steps in applying the RAM are shown in Figure 1. First, a detailed literature review is performed to synthesise the latest available scientific evidence on the procedure to be rated. At the same time, a list of specific clinical scenarios or "indications" is produced in the form of a matrix which categorises patients who might present for the procedure in question in terms of their symptoms, past medical history and the results of relevant diagnostic tests. These indications are grouped into "chapters" based on the primary presenting symptom leading to a patient's being referred for treatment or considered for a particular procedure. An example of a specific indication for coronary revascularization in the chapter on "Chronic Stable Angina" is:

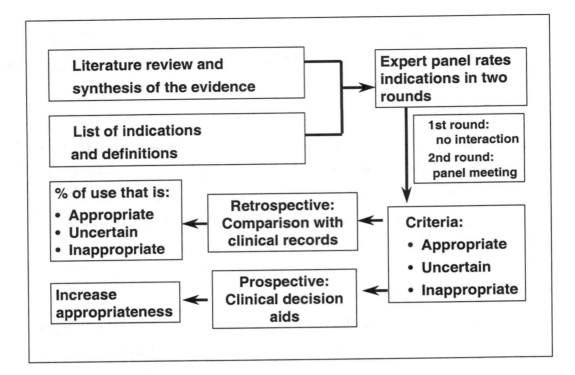

Figure 1: The RAND/UCLA Appropriateness Method

A patient with severe angina (class III/IV) in spite of optimal medical therapy, who has 2-vessel disease without involvement of the proximal left anterior descending artery, an ejection fraction of between 30 and 50%, a very positive stress test, and who is at low to moderate surgical risk.

A panel of experts is identified, often based on recommendations from the relevant medical societies. The literature review and the list of indications, together with a list of definitions for all terms used in the indications list, are sent to the members of this panel. For each indication, the panel members rate the benefit-to-harm ratio of the procedure on a scale of 1 to 9, where 1 means that the expected harms greatly outweigh the expected benefits, and 9 means that the expected benefits greatly outweigh the expected harms. A middle rating of 5 can mean either that the harms and benefits are about equal or that the rater cannot make the judgement for the patient described in the indication.

The panellists rate each of the indications twice, in a two-round "modified Delphi" process. In the first round, the ratings are made individually at home, with no interaction among panellists. In the second round, the panel members meet for 1-2 days under the leadership of a moderator experienced in using the method. Each panellist receives an individualised document showing the distribution of all the experts' first round ratings, together with his/her own specific ratings. During the meeting, panellists discuss the ratings, focusing on areas of disagreement, and are given the opportunity to modify the original list of indications and/or definitions, if desired. After discussing each chapter of the list of indications, they re-rate each indication individually. No attempt is made to force the panel to consensus. Instead, the two-round process is designed to sort out whether discrepant ratings are due to real clinical disagreement over the use of the procedure ("real" disagreement) or to fatigue or misunderstanding ("artifactual" disagreement).

Finally, each indication is classified as "appropriate," "uncertain" or "inappropriate" for the procedure under review in accordance with the panellists' median score and the level of disagreement among the panellists. Indications with median scores in the 1-3 range are classified as inappropriate, those in the 4-6 range as uncertain, and those in the 7-9 range as appropriate. However, all indications rated "with disagreement," whatever the median, are classified as uncertain. "Disagreement" here basically means a lack of consensus, either because there is polarisation of the group or because judgements are spread over the entire 1 to 9 rating scale. As discussed in Chapter 8, various alternative definitions for disagreement have been used throughout the history of the RAM.

Appropriateness studies sometimes categorise levels of agreement further to identify indications rated "with agreement" and those rated with "indeterminate" agreement (neither agreement nor disagreement). Depending on how the appropriateness criteria are to be used, it may sometimes be desirable to identify those indications rated with greater or lesser levels of agreement.

If necessity criteria are also to be developed, a third round of ratings takes place, usually by mail, in which panellists are asked to rate the necessity of those indications that have been classified as appropriate by the panel. The RAM definition of necessity (Kahan et al., 1994a) is that:

- The procedure is appropriate, i.e., the health benefits exceed the risks by a sufficient margin to make it worth doing.
- It would be improper care not to offer the procedure to a patient.
- There is a reasonable chance that the procedure will benefit the patient.
- The magnitude of the expected benefit is not small.

All four of the preceding criteria must be met for a procedure to be considered as necessary for a particular indication. To determine necessity, indications rated appropriate by the panel are presented for a further rating of necessity. This rating is also done on a scale of 1 to 9, where 1 means the procedure is clearly not necessary and 9 means it clearly is necessary. If panellists disagree in their necessity ratings or if the median is less than 7, then the indication is judged as "appropriate but not necessary." Only appropriate indications with a necessity rating of 7 or more without disagreement are judged "necessary."

Comparison with Other Group Judgement Methods

The RAM is only one of several methods that have been developed to identify the collective opinion of experts (Fink et al., 1984). Although it is often called a "consensus method," it does not really belong in that category, because its objective is to detect when the experts agree, rather than to obtain a consensus among them. It is based on the so-called "Delphi method," developed at RAND in the 1950s as a tool to predict the future, which was applied to political-military, technological and economic topics (Linstone et al., 1975). The Delphi process has since also come to be used in a variety of health and medical settings. The method generally involves multiple rounds, in which a questionnaire is sent to a group of experts who answer the questions anonymously. The results of the survey are then tabulated and reported back to the group, and each person is asked to answer the questionnaire again. This iterative process continues until there is a convergence of opinion on the subject or no further substantial changes in the replies are elicited.

The RAM is sometimes miscast as an example of the Nominal Group Technique (NGT). NGT is a highly structured process in which participants are brought together and asked to write down all their ideas on a particular subject. The moderator asks each person to briefly describe the most important idea on his or her list, and continues around the table until everyone's ideas have been listed. After discussion of each topic, participants are asked to individually rank order or rate their judgement of the item's importance on a numerical scale. Different mathematical techniques are used to aggregate the results. The RAM, unlike the NGT, begins with a highly structured list of clinical indications, and the discussion is tightly linked to the basic measurement of appropriateness.

A third group judgement method is the Consensus Development Conference. The U.S. National Institutes of Health (NIH) have a mandate to evaluate and disseminate information about health care technologies and biomedical research (Kanouse, 1989). To this end, they have developed what are known as NIH Consensus Conferences, which bring together a wide variety of participants, including physicians, researchers and consumers, who are charged with developing a mutually acceptable consensus statement to answer specific, pre-defined questions about the topic. This process includes conducting a literature review, summarising the current state of knowledge, presentations by experts and advocates, and audience discussion. These conferences frequently last 2 or more days, and do not end until the participants have agreed on a written statement. Many European countries have developed their own versions of Consensus Conferences.

At its centre, the RAM is a modified Delphi method that, unlike the original Delphi, provides panellists with the opportunity to discuss their judgements between the rating rounds. Contrary to the fears of the original developers of Delphi, experience with the RAM and the contemporaneous literature on group processes both indicate that the potential for bias in a face-to-face group can be largely controlled by effective group leadership (e.g., Kahan et al., 1994b). Thus, while panellists receive feedback on the group's responses, as is done in the classic Delphi method, they have a chance to discuss their answers in a face-to-face meeting, similar to the NGT and NIH Consensus Conferences.

CHAPTER 2. SELECTING A TOPIC

Most studies using the RAM have focused on medical or surgical procedures that meet some or all of the following criteria:

- Procedures that are used frequently
- Procedures that are associated with a substantial amount of morbidity and/or mortality
- Procedures that consume significant resources
- Procedures with wide variations among geographic areas in rates of use
- Procedures whose use is controversial.

The greater the extent to which these criteria are met, the greater is the potential impact of applying the appropriateness criteria.

Researchers may decide to select a particular topic either because of their own interest in the subject, in which case they will usually need to develop a proposal and submit it to potential funding sources, or because the topic is identified for them by an external agency. In either case, the first step is to determine whether previous appropriateness studies have been done on the topic (see Table 1). If they have, it can be very helpful to contact the research group involved to obtain a copy of the list of indications, literature review and other documents used in the previous project. Annex I contains a list of the institutions involved in the European Union BIOMED Concerted Action on the appropriateness of medical and surgical procedures, together with the names of the persons representing each institution.

An important aspect to consider in selecting a topic is the quality of the scientific evidence available. Because the RAM is a technique for extrapolating from an evidence base to a larger set of indications, it is dependent upon that initial base of evidence. If the quality of the evidence is low—that is, there is little evidence from well-conducted randomised clinical trials—the reliability of the panel process is likely to be lower. For example, a US study found lower levels of agreement among three randomly selected panels of experts that rated the appropriateness of indications for hysterectomy than among three similar panels rating indications for coronary revascularization, where the evidence base was much stronger (Shekelle et al., 1998b).

Table 1. Some Procedures Studied Using the RAND/UCLA Appropriateness Method[a]

Procedure	Country
Abdominal aortic aneurysm surgery	United States
Benign prostatic hyperplasia (prostatectomy)	Spain, United Kingdom
Benign prostatic hyperplasia (comparison of treatments)	The Netherlands, European panel
Breast cancer (limited surgery)	Italy
Carotid endarterectomy	United States
Cataract surgery	Italy, United States
Cholecystectomy	Israel, United Kingdom, United States
Coronary angiography	Canada, Spain, Sweden, Switzerland, United Kingdom, United States
Coronary revascularization (PTCA and CABG)	Canada, Germany, Italy, the Netherlands, Spain, Sweden, Switzerland, United Kingdom, United States, European panel
Depression	The Netherlands
Endoscopy (upper and lower gastrointestinal)	Switzerland, United States, European panel
Haemophilia (treatment with Factor VIII)	Spain
Hip replacement	Spain
Hysterectomy	Sweden, Switzerland, United States
Laminectomy	Switzerland, United States
Preoperative use of recombinant erythropoietin	United States
Spinal manipulation for lower back pain	United States
Tympanostomy tubes	United States

[a] See Van het Loo and Kahan (1999) for references to each of these studies.

Most studies to date have focused on specific procedures—either diagnostic or therapeutic—but some have also taken a more comprehensive approach by studying the management of a particular disease or condition, such as ischemic heart disease or benign prostatic hyperplasia.

CHAPTER 3. REVIEW AND SYNTHESIS OF THE LITERATURE

Purpose

Fundamental to any appropriateness study is a critical review of the literature summarising the scientific evidence available on the procedure under review. Such a review is necessary to ensure that all panel members have access to the same body of evidence, and as a resource to resolve any disagreements that may arise during the meeting which can be addressed by reference to specific studies.

Much has been written about literature reviews, and their quality has increased considerably with the advent of the Cochrane Collaboration, which attempts to produce reliable, systematic reviews of the effects of health care interventions (Chalmers, 1993). However, the objectives of a literature review developed for an appropriateness study are somewhat different: a Cochrane review is generally limited to scientific evidence from randomised controlled trials or similarly methodologically rigorous research, whereas an appropriateness review includes the best available evidence, which may not always meet Cochrane standards. Cochrane reviewers use a precise, standardised methodology to review potential articles, with strict inclusion and exclusion criteria to assure that only evidence from well-conducted randomised controlled trials is included. Meta-analysis is frequently used, in which the results of different studies are combined to increase statistical power. Literature reviews for appropriateness studies are typically less strict in their inclusion criteria, as the objective is to produce a synthesis of all the information available on a particular topic; where evidence from controlled trials is lacking, they may well include lower quality evidence from, for example, cohort studies or case series. Our view, in brief, is that a systematic review such as done within the Cochrane Collaboration, if supplemented by other sources, is a good way to conduct a RAM literature review.

While it is not the purpose of this manual to describe in detail how to carry out a literature review, as this has been well documented elsewhere (e.g., Goodman, 1993), we present a brief review of the steps to be followed in producing this document.

Search Methodology

The literature review should include a precise description of the questions to be addressed, the search methodology used, and the criteria followed in selecting and classifying articles. Typically, the review begins with a MEDLINE search—though other databases may also be included, for instance, the Cochrane Library when looking for systematic reviews of randomised trials—for all relevant articles about the efficacy, risks and utilisation of the procedure of interest. Information on costs may also be included, although the panel will specifically be instructed not to take cost considerations into account when making their appropriateness ratings. The search strategy used [including specification of Medical Subject Heading (MESH) and non-MESH terms] should be documented in the final report to help the reader judge if the literature review is based on an adequate body of evidence. As is well known, however, even the most carefully planned MEDLINE search will not identify all articles related with these subjects, therefore it is also useful to review manually the reference lists of selected articles. Review articles and meta-analyses are good sources for additional references. Abstracts of studies that have not been published as complete articles (e.g., conference abstracts) are not included. Experts in the field may also be asked about possible omissions in the reference list. Obviously, a very sensitive search strategy will lack specificity, therefore some restrictions may be applied, for example: language (limited to English), year of publication (last 10 years), abstract available, and so on. Care should be taken in applying restrictions, however, as they may produce a biased assessment of the literature.

If a previous review of the literature is available on the topic at hand, this can provide a good basis for the new review. Depending on what new developments have occurred since the last review, however, it may be better to do an entirely new review than to include a large amount of data from studies that are largely outdated. High quality systematic reviews, if they are available, may constitute a substantial contribution to the available evidence.

Selection and Classification of Articles

A system should be used to classify articles according to the study methodology, which is usually a good indicator of the quality of the evidence produced. There are many such classification systems, for example, in order of decreasing strength of evidence:

1) Large randomised controlled trials

2) Small randomised controlled trials

3) Non-randomised trials with contemporaneous controls

4) Non-randomised trials with historical controls

5) Cohort studies

6) Case-control studies

7) Cross-sectional studies

8) Surveillance (e.g., using databases or registries)

9) Series of consecutive cases

Other classification systems exist; what they all have in common is that the greatest weight is given to evidence from randomised controlled trials. Where this is not available, or is of questionable quality, evidence from lower quality studies may also be cited. Scales have been developed to rate the quality of randomised controlled trials, and these may also be applied.

Synthesising the Evidence

Once the articles to be included are selected, the data must be integrated and organised into a final report. If feasible, it will be helpful to the panellists to organise the literature review using the same chapter headings as in the list of indications (see Chapter 4, "Structure of the List of Indications"). In discussing a particular article, mention should be made of the type of study (e.g., "double blind randomised controlled trial," "observational study") to give the reader an idea of the quality of the evidence supporting its results. Some reviews may also include a summary measure of the quality of the evidence supporting a conclusion based on different studies (level A, B, C or D evidence, for example.) Finally, mention should also be made of areas in which studies have yielded contradictory or uncertain results.

Where possible, "evidence tables" summarising the data from multiple studies should be included in the literature review. For example, a 1998 literature review of gastrointestinal endoscopy showed summary results of complication rates in patients undergoing diagnostic colonoscopy (Table 2). Such tables can be difficult to develop because studies frequently differ in their definitions of different events, follow-up time, and so on. They are worth the effort, however, because they provide a good way to help the reader quickly compare the main outcomes of different studies.

Table 2. Complication Rates in Patients Undergoing Diagnostic Colonoscopy

Reference	No. of Procedures	Mortality	Morbidity				
			Total	Bleeding	Perforation	Other	Surgery required
Kahn	85,545	0.02	0.25	0.03	0.20	0.03	0.05
Macrea	5,000	0.06	—	0.02	0.06	—	—
Gilbert	4,713	0	—	0.11	0.17	—	—
Hahr-Gama	3,256	0	—	0	0.06	—	—
Reiertsen	3,538	0	0.14	0.03	—	0.11	—
Waye	1,320	0	0	0	0	0.3	—

Source: Bochud et al., 1998.

Resources Required

It is difficult to quantify exactly how many persons should work on the literature review and how long it will take, though one can generally assume the two are inversely proportional. The amount of resources required will depend on the complexity of the subject to be reviewed, the amount of literature available, and the time period to be covered, among other factors. Ideally, one person should have experience in bibliographic searches, while the other persons should have some knowledge of how to rate the quality of scientific articles and synthesise information from different sources. Research proposals incorporating the appropriateness method should budget sufficient funds for this step. If it is not possible to pay for this work, the persons responsible for researching and writing the literature review should be freed from other tasks during a specified time. Experience from other studies has shown that a minimum of 6 months of total effort is required to produce an adequate literature review if no previous literature review is available.

CHAPTER 4. DEVELOPING THE LIST OF INDICATIONS AND DEFINITIONS

Characteristics of the List of Indications

Concurrent with the summary of the evidence emerging from the literature review, a list of the hypothetical clinical scenarios or "indications" to be rated by the panel is developed. The purpose of the list of indications is to classify patients in terms of the clinical variables physicians take into account in deciding whether to recommend a particular procedure. This list is the basic working document used in the panel process. The list of indications should be 1) comprehensive, so as to include a wide range of patients who might present to a physician for the procedure under review[*]; 2) mutually exclusive, so that no patient can be classified in more than one indication; 3) homogeneous, so that the decision on the appropriateness of the procedure would apply equally to all persons classified in the particular indication; and 4) manageable, so that panellists can rate all the indications in a reasonable length of time. In previous appropriateness studies, the list of indications has ranged from about 200 (cholecystectomy) to over 3000 (cataract surgery) indications. Any more than 2000 indications is generally agreed to be difficult to manage.

The list of indications—along with concise and explicit definitions of all terms used in the list—is developed by clinicians who are experienced in the procedure under study, in collaboration with members of the research team who understand the appropriateness methodology. If the procedure has already been the subject of an appropriateness study, it can be helpful to begin with an indications list developed previously and modify it so that it is consistent with the way clinical decisions are made in a particular country, region or institution. For example, a number of countries have now carried out studies on the appropriateness of PTCA and CABG. The indications lists used in each study are similar to the one first developed for use in the United States, but have been changed to reflect the factors taken into account by cardiologists and cardiovascular surgeons in each country, as well as new scientific evidence. For example, different boundaries have been

---

[*] Early RAM studies tried to include almost all patients who might present for a procedure; more recently, however, many studies have focused on indications that are known to represent substantial numbers of real patients.

established for the ejection fraction categories and varying numbers of stress test categories have been used.

Structure of the List of Indications

The indications categorise patients in terms of their personal characteristics (e.g., age, gender when relevant), symptoms, medical history, and diagnostic test results. Typically, the list is divided into chapters, in accordance with the patient's main presenting symptom, and each chapter is subdivided by the different variables used. The variables are listed in rows and columns so that most or all possible combinations are included. This approach may result in the inclusion of some (or many) combinations of variables that do not actually occur in clinical practice, or that occur only rarely. However, many studies continue to use this approach because 1) it is difficult to identify beforehand which indications actually occur in clinical practice; 2) the rating process may be easier when a consistent logic is used in listing the identifications; and 3) the complete list is amenable to certain kinds of statistical analysis. Figure 2 shows the main variables used in one list of indications for coronary revascularization.

Figure 3 shows a page from the "Chronic Stable Angina" chapter of the list of indications used for the Spanish panel on the appropriateness of coronary revascularization. This figure gives an idea of how the different variables were combined to create the rating structure. Indication number 1 on this list describes a patient with chronic stable angina which is severe (class III/IV) in spite of optimal medical therapy, who has left main disease, a left ventricular ejection fraction greater than 50%, and who is at low or moderate surgical risk, for whom the panel is considering the appropriateness of coronary revascularization compared to continued medical therapy. This figure also illustrates the rating forms used by the panellists.

In preparing the chapters, care should be taken not to make them too complicated. Five or six levels of variables are about the maximum per chapter, as a larger number may prove difficult to handle. If additional variables are needed to adequately describe patients, the chapter might be split into two by adding a clinically relevant variable, for example, chronic vs. acute, first vs. subsequent episodes, and so on.

Major presenting symptom: (CHAPTER headings)	Asymptomatic Chronic stable angina Unstable angina Acute myocardial infarction Post myocardial infarction Near sudden death Palliative PTCA Emergency CABG
Severity of coronary artery disease:	Left main Three vessels Two vessels with proximal left anterior descending (PLAD) involvement Two vessels without PLAD involvement One vessel (PLAD) One vessel (any except PLAD)
Angina Class	Mild or Moderate (Canadian Cardiovascular Society class I/II) Severe (class III/IV)
Left ventricular ejection fraction:	> 50% > 30$\leq$50% > 20$\leq$30%
Stress test results:	Positive Negative Indeterminate or not done
Medical therapy:	Optimal Sub-optimal
Surgical risk:	Low or moderate High

Figure 2. Variables in List of Indications for Rating the Appropriateness of Coronary Revascularization. Spanish Panel, December 1996

Another example of an indications matrix is shown in Figure 4. This list was developed for a European panel rating the appropriateness of upper and lower gastrointestinal endoscopy. The first indication on this list refers to a patient under 45 years of age with a first or second episode of uncomplicated dyspepsia, who has either not been previously evaluated by upper GI endoscopy or the results of a previous investigation are not known, has not been tested for *Helicobacter pylori*, is not receiving acid lowering medications, and whose symptoms have resolved. The next chapter in this list of indications is identical, except that it refers to patients with recurrent episodes of uncomplicated dyspepsia; this is an example of how a chapter can be split into two if the variables become too difficult to handle.

CHAPTER 2

	Low/Moderate Surgical Risk		High Surgical Risk		
CHRONIC STABLE ANGINA	Appropriateness of Med. Ther. - Revasc.	Appropriateness of PTCA - CABG	Appropriateness of Med. Ther. - Revasc.	Appropriateness of PTCA - CABG	Indic. No.
A. PATIENT HAS SEVERE ANGINA (CLASS III/IV) IN SPITE OF OPTIMAL MEDICAL THERAPY					
1. Left main disease					
LVEF a) >50%	1 2 3 4 5 6 7 8 9	1 2 3 4 5 6 7 8 9	1 2 3 4 5 6 7 8 9	1 2 3 4 5 6 7 8 9	(1-4)
b) >30% ≤50%	1 2 3 4 5 6 7 8 9	1 2 3 4 5 6 7 8 9	1 2 3 4 5 6 7 8 9	1 2 3 4 5 6 7 8 9	(5-8)
c) >20% ≤30%	1 2 3 4 5 6 7 8 9	1 2 3 4 5 6 7 8 9	1 2 3 4 5 6 7 8 9	1 2 3 4 5 6 7 8 9	(9-12)
2. Three vessel disease					
LVEF a) >50%	1 2 3 4 5 6 7 8 9	1 2 3 4 5 6 7 8 9	1 2 3 4 5 6 7 8 9	1 2 3 4 5 6 7 8 9	(13-16)
b) >30% ≤50%	1 2 3 4 5 6 7 8 9	1 2 3 4 5 6 7 8 9	1 2 3 4 5 6 7 8 9	1 2 3 4 5 6 7 8 9	(17-20)
c) >20% ≤30%	1 2 3 4 5 6 7 8 9	1 2 3 4 5 6 7 8 9	1 2 3 4 5 6 7 8 9	1 2 3 4 5 6 7 8 9	(21-24)
3. Two vessel disease with proximal left anterior descending (PLAD) involvement					
LVEF a) >50%	1 2 3 4 5 6 7 8 9	1 2 3 4 5 6 7 8 9	1 2 3 4 5 6 7 8 9	1 2 3 4 5 6 7 8 9	(25-28)
b) >30% ≤50%	1 2 3 4 5 6 7 8 9	1 2 3 4 5 6 7 8 9	1 2 3 4 5 6 7 8 9	1 2 3 4 5 6 7 8 9	(29-32)
c) >20% ≤30%	1 2 3 4 5 6 7 8 9	1 2 3 4 5 6 7 8 9	1 2 3 4 5 6 7 8 9	1 2 3 4 5 6 7 8 9	(33-36)
4. Two vessel disease without proximal left anterior descending (PLAD) involvement					
LVEF a) >50%	1 2 3 4 5 6 7 8 9	1 2 3 4 5 6 7 8 9	1 2 3 4 5 6 7 8 9	1 2 3 4 5 6 7 8 9	(37-40)
b) >30% ≤50%	1 2 3 4 5 6 7 8 9	1 2 3 4 5 6 7 8 9	1 2 3 4 5 6 7 8 9	1 2 3 4 5 6 7 8 9	(41-44)
c) >20% ≤30%	1 2 3 4 5 6 7 8 9	1 2 3 4 5 6 7 8 9	1 2 3 4 5 6 7 8 9	1 2 3 4 5 6 7 8 9	(45-48)
5. One vessel disease (PLAD)					
LVEF a) >50%	1 2 3 4 5 6 7 8 9	1 2 3 4 5 6 7 8 9	1 2 3 4 5 6 7 8 9	1 2 3 4 5 6 7 8 9	(49-52)
b) >30% ≤50%	1 2 3 4 5 6 7 8 9	1 2 3 4 5 6 7 8 9	1 2 3 4 5 6 7 8 9	1 2 3 4 5 6 7 8 9	(53-56)
c) >20% ≤30%	1 2 3 4 5 6 7 8 9	1 2 3 4 5 6 7 8 9	1 2 3 4 5 6 7 8 9	1 2 3 4 5 6 7 8 9	(57-60)
6. One vessel disease (any except PLAD)					
LVEF a) >50%	1 2 3 4 5 6 7 8 9	1 2 3 4 5 6 7 8 9	1 2 3 4 5 6 7 8 9	1 2 3 4 5 6 7 8 9	(49-52)
b) >30% ≤50%	1 2 3 4 5 6 7 8 9	1 2 3 4 5 6 7 8 9	1 2 3 4 5 6 7 8 9	1 2 3 4 5 6 7 8 9	(53-56)
c) >20% ≤30%	1 2 3 4 5 6 7 8 9	1 2 3 4 5 6 7 8 9	1 2 3 4 5 6 7 8 9	1 2 3 4 5 6 7 8 9	(57-60)

1 = Highly inappropriate; 9 = Highly appropriate

Figure 3. Sample Indications List from Spanish Coronary Revascularization Panel, December 1996

Panelist1; round1; page 1

CHAPTER 1
Upper GI Endoscopy
Uncomplicated Dyspepsia:
1ST OR 2ND EPISODE(S)

	Less than 45 years old		45 years old or older		
	NSAID	No NSAID	NSAID	No NSAID	
A. No previous investigation or previous investigation with results unknown					
1. No HP test, no empiric acid lowering treatment					
a. Symptoms resolved	1 2 3 4 5 6 7 8 9	1 2 3 4 5 6 7 8 9	1 2 3 4 5 6 7 8 9	1 2 3 4 5 6 7 8 9	(1-4)
b. Symptoms not resolved	1 2 3 4 5 6 7 8 9	1 2 3 4 5 6 7 8 9	1 2 3 4 5 6 7 8 9	1 2 3 4 5 6 7 8 9	(5-8)
2. No HP test, empiric acid lowering treatment given					
a. Symptoms resolved	1 2 3 4 5 6 7 8 9	1 2 3 4 5 6 7 8 9	1 2 3 4 5 6 7 8 9	1 2 3 4 5 6 7 8 9	(9-12)
b. Symptoms not resolved	1 2 3 4 5 6 7 8 9	1 2 3 4 5 6 7 8 9	1 2 3 4 5 6 7 8 9	1 2 3 4 5 6 7 8 9	(13-16)
3. HP test negative, no empiric acid lowering treatment					
a. Symptoms resolved	1 2 3 4 5 6 7 8 9	1 2 3 4 5 6 7 8 9	1 2 3 4 5 6 7 8 9	1 2 3 4 5 6 7 8 9	(17-20)
b. Symptoms not resolved	1 2 3 4 5 6 7 8 9	1 2 3 4 5 6 7 8 9	1 2 3 4 5 6 7 8 9	1 2 3 4 5 6 7 8 9	(21-24)

Appropriateness scale: 1 = extremely inappropriate, 5 = uncertain, 9 = extremely appropriate

Figure 4. Sample Indications List from European Gastrointestinal Endoscopy Panel, November 1998

Throughout the process of developing the list of indications, it is helpful to ask such questions as: Could this patient be classified in more than one cell of the matrix? Are there any other clinical variables that physicians usually take into account in deciding when to apply this procedure? Are there other types of patients for whom this procedure might be considered? If the list turns out to be very long (numbering more than 2000 indications), consideration might be given to reducing its length by concentrating on those indications that represent a substantial number of patients (if this is known) or by narrowing the goals of the study to a smaller group of patients.

Modifying the List of Indications (Before the Panel Meeting)

After the initial indication matrix is created, it should be carefully reviewed to see if there are some sections that are clearly unnecessary or do not make clinical sense. For example, knowledge of ejection fraction may be important in deciding whether or not to revascularize patients with most types of vessel disease, but it may not matter if the patient has left main disease. If this is clearly the case, there is no point in asking panellists to rate each category of ejection fraction for these patients. Similarly, knowledge of the patient's age group may be important for some clinical decisions, but not for others. If there is any doubt, however, as to whether a particular variable might be relevant to the clinical decision at hand, it is probably better to leave it in. If the results of the first round ratings show that panellists do not take the variable into consideration, it is easy to collapse categories during the second round [see "Modifying the List of Indications (During the Panel Meeting)" in Chapter 7].

It is useful to have as much input as possible when developing the list of indications. If time and resources permit, the list could be sent to the panellists before they do the actual ratings, to give them a chance to see the proposed structure and suggest possible changes. If this is done, the panel moderator or a member of the research team should follow-up by telephone to elicit each panellist's suggestions of how the structure of the list could be improved. If panellists agree on major revisions, new rating sheets could then be prepared. Alternatively, the research team may contact the panellists between the first and second rounds of ratings to discuss the indication structure. Once again, if panellists agree on major revisions, new rating sheets could be prepared for the panel meeting.

Another interesting approach was used during a Dutch study of treatment for benign prostatic hyperplasia (BPH). A "round zero" panel meeting was organised in which the RAND/UCLA method was described, and in which the panel discussed the population, treatments and diagnostic parameters to be included. The advantages of this approach are that:

- It gives the panel members a chance to become familiar with the RAND/UCLA method, thereby facilitating the rating of the initial list of indications.

- It increases the efficiency of the panel process by avoiding much of the discussion about definitions, diagnostic parameters and cut-off points that usually takes place after the first round of ratings.

- It contributes to the development of a team atmosphere, builds confidence and helps create a positive environment for future work.

The Dutch investigators found that this approach resulted in very low levels of disagreement in the first-round ratings. A more recent study of the use of Factor VIII in the treatment of haemophilia also held a round zero meeting to facilitate creation of the list of indications. Depending on the travel time involved, however, this extra meeting may result in considerable additional costs.

Definitions of Terms

The persons who develop the indications list must also write concise and explicit definitions of each term used in the list. Panellists cannot be sure they are all rating the same indication unless they have a precise definition of each term. Thus, as important as the list of indications is an accompanying document defining each term used in the list. These definitions must take into account how clinical decisions are made in the particular setting where the method is being applied. How physicians define a "positive stress test," or "high surgical risk," for instance, may vary from country to country. Having the definitions on hand during the meeting where the second round ratings are done is also important. Some disagreements during the panel meeting may be resolved by the panellist's realisation that they are not all using the same definitions. What, for example, constitutes "moderate limitation of functional capacity" for a panel considering the appropriateness of different devices for hip replacement? The moderator may want to read the definition if he or she thinks this may be the cause of disagreement, to be sure everyone is thinking of the same patient. Of course, panellists are free to modify the definitions during the meeting if they can agree on mutually acceptable wording. If this is the case, the moderator may want to write the new definition on a blackboard or flipchart to make sure everyone is clear about the new definition to be used.

Figures 5 and 6 show sample sections from the lists of definitions developed for appropriateness studies of gastrointestinal endoscopy and laminectomy, respectively.

CHAPTER 1 and CHAPTER 2: Uncomplicated dyspepsia

Dyspepsia
Is defined as pain or discomfort in the abdomen, including nausea, vomiting, early satiety, epigastric fullness but not heartburn or dysphagia. Furthermore, isolated heartburn or regurgitation are dealt with in chapter 3.

Uncomplicated dyspepsia
Dyspepsia without alarm symptoms.

Alarm symptoms
One or more of the following: melena, weight loss, anaemia, hematemesis, esophageal dysphagia (definitions of these terms are in chapter 6).

Episode of dyspepsia
Minimum duration to be considered as an episode: 7 days (1 week).
Recurrent episodes: ≥3 episodes, as opposed to first or second episode.
Time interval to define the onset of a new episode: 1 month free of symptoms without treatment.

Eradication treatment
Treatment regimen composed of two antibiotics and a proton-pump inhibitor or an H2 blocker with an eradication rate supposed to exceed 90%.

Helicobacter test
According to the situation, either
- non-endoscopic test (serology, Carbon 13 breath-test), or
- endoscopic test (urease test, histology, culture)

Figure 5. Sample Definitions from European Gastrointestinal Endoscopy Panel, November 1998

Laminectomy: Includes unilateral and bilateral laminectomy, with discectomy and open microsdiscectomy: does not include percutaneous procedures, nor spinal fusion.

Note: A laminectomy proposed three months or more since a previous laminectomy uses the indications in chapters 1-9.

The laminectomy indications also apply with recurrent sciatica.

SYMPTOMS

1. Sciatica or cruralgia

Pain in the posterior or lateral aspect of one lower extremity distal to the knee (sciatica) or anterior portion of one thigh (cruralgia).

In patients with both back and leg pain, the leg pain must predominate. If the magnitude of the leg pain is similar to the magnitude of the back pain, it is considered sciatica if the pain is in a dermatomal pattern.

- Acute: Symptoms present for less than 6 weeks.
- Subacute: Symptoms present for 6 weeks to 6 months.
- Chronic: Symptoms present for more than 6 months.

2. Symptoms of Central Spinal Stenosis

Neurogenic claudication (unilateral or bilateral lower limb pain, weakness or paresthesia made worse by walking and relieved by sitting or bending forward).

3. Symptoms of Lateral Spinal Stenosis

Unilateral lower extremity pain in a radicular distribution; or numbness, paresthesia or weakness corresponding to a radicular distribution; includes sciatica.

Figure 6. Sample Definitions from Swiss Back Surgery Panel, 1995

CHAPTER 5. THE EXPERT PANEL

Panel Composition

The composition of the panel is important. Some panels have represented a single medical speciality, such as urology, but most have been multidisciplinary, including those who perform the procedure, physicians in related specialities and sometimes primary care providers. Most users of the RAND/UCLA method recommend using multidisciplinary panels to better reflect the variety of specialities that are actually involved in patient treatment decisions. Previous studies have shown that, in general, those who perform a procedure tend to rate higher on the appropriateness scale than those who do not, with the result that more indications are rated appropriate by the panel than when multiple specialities are represented (Kahan et al., 1995).

The decision as to which speciality or specialities to include will depend on the particular procedure under study and the way clinical decisions are made in each country. In studies of the appropriateness of PTCA and CABG, a United States panel had three cardiothoracic surgeons, three invasive cardiologists, one non-invasive cardiologist, and two internists. A Swedish panel was similarly composed, but also included an epidemiologist, while a 12-member Spanish panel was made up of 4 cardiothoracic surgeons, 4 invasive cardiologists and 4 non-invasive cardiologists. In Spain it was not considered necessary to include internists because they are not involved in these kinds of treatment decisions. In Switzerland, neurosurgeons were heavily represented in the panel convened to develop appropriateness criteria for surgery of lumbar disk hernia because they perform many related surgical interventions. The Dutch panel on treatment for benign prostatic hyperplasia (BPH) included only urologists (from both university hospitals and general clinics), because in The Netherlands the choice between invasive and less invasive treatment modalities for BPH is not made by the general practitioner.

Panel Nominations

Nominations for panel members may be solicited from a variety of sources: speciality societies, universities, individuals. It is usually a good idea to enlist the support of medical societies of physicians in the relevant disciplines by requesting them to nominate potential panellists, not least because societies that have participated in the process are more likely to support the resulting recommendations. Multiple nominations should be solicited, and the curriculum vitae of the potential panellists should be carefully reviewed. The main selection criteria to be considered are acknowledged leadership in the panel member's speciality, absence of conflicts of interest, geographic diversity, and diversity of practice setting. Panellists should not be chosen just because they are easily accessible or to keep transportation costs to a minimum. The project leader may also want to check informally with people who know potential panel members to have an idea if they are likely to work well with their colleagues in this kind of process. Highly domineering individuals, or those who are known to have rigid views on the subject matter, are probably to be avoided.

If the panel is to include people from different countries who will need to speak a common language (e.g., English), it is important to assure that the candidates have good oral comprehension and are comfortable speaking that language.

How Many Members?

The earliest RAND appropriateness panels were composed of 9 members. There is nothing magical about this number, though, and other studies have used panels ranging from 7 to 15 members. The rationale behind the 9-member RAND panels was that they were large enough to permit diversity of representation while still being small enough to allow everyone to be involved in the group discussion. While this is true, some variation around that number will preserve these desirable group qualities. The number 9 somehow acquired a "magical" property—perhaps because the original statistical treatments of the panel results were defined for that panel size and subsequent studies employed that number to avoid having to modify definitions. However, it can be difficult to assure that exactly 9 panellists participate in the second round: if only 9 are invited, it is quite possible that at least 1 will be a "no-show," and if more are invited, they may all show up. This has been a problem in some previous panels, requiring the research group to come up with new, and not necessarily common, definitions of disagreement for panels of fewer than or more than 9 persons. To resolve these kinds of problems, work is currently being done on the development of a new statistic to define disagreement (and agreement) that will apply to any size panel (see Chapter 8). In summary, then, panels can be of any size that permits sufficient diversity (a minimum of 7), while ensuring that all have a chance to participate (probably a maximum of 15). The best choice within this range depends on the desired geographic and disciplinary representation on the panel.

Motivation to Participate

Panellists are generally honoured to be asked to serve on an expert panel, since it indicates they are respected by their colleagues and their opinion is valued. In the United States, panellists have often been given a small honorarium for their time and effort. If the research budget so allows, it may be desirable to offer a token payment to panel members, though experience in several European countries has shown that panel members participate willingly and enthusiastically without such remuneration.

Another factor that may encourage panel participation is the meeting itself. The panellists typically enjoy the collegiality of the process and the meeting is usually held in a pleasant location. Insofar as possible, however, it is better to avoid conducting a panel where many of the panellists work, since they may be distracted by patient or other job demands. All major expenses (hotel, meals and, if possible, travel costs) should be paid "up front" by the project, rather than asking panellists to advance money for these purposes. In addition, any incidental costs born by the panellists (taxis, meals outside the meeting times) should be promptly reimbursed. The added expense of the rare panellist who abuses the system is more than compensated for by the general good will achieved.

Contacts with Panellists

After selecting the initial list of candidates from among the nominations of specialist societies and other sources, someone from the research team should make a preliminary contact by phone to establish their interest and availability. Those who express a desire to participate in the panel process may be asked to send a curriculum vitae to help the research group evaluate their contributions to their field of expertise. The person conducting these initial interviews should let panellists know that contacts are being made with experts from a variety of clinical specialities (or geographic regions or practice settings or whatever selection criteria are being used) and that not all persons contacted will be selected. A delicate approach is needed to avoid giving offence to those who are not asked to serve on the panel.

Once candidate panellists are selected, each should receive a letter explaining what the RAND/UCLA appropriateness method is and how it will be applied to the procedure under study. A calendar might be supplied with this letter, asking them to indicate dates they could be available for the panel meeting. Alternatively—and more effectively—firm dates can be chosen well ahead of time; most panellists can then enter these dates into their calendars before competing activities make finding a date impossible. When there are many potential panellists who are largely equally desirable, a quasi-random selection strategy is to set firm dates and let invitees accept on the basis of their availability on those dates. The project leader and/or co-ordinator should let panellists know when and where they can be located in case the panellists have any questions about the process.

The panel meeting is usually scheduled for 1 to 2 days. Once the dates have been confirmed, all panellists need to be notified immediately so they can block out these days on their calendars. Meetings are often held on a Friday-Saturday to minimise interference with the work week (and to take advantage of cheaper airfares).

When the panel documents (that is, the literature review, list of indications, definitions and instructions) are ready, they should be mailed to the panellists with a letter of introduction listing the enclosures and explaining how they are to be used. Stamped, pre-addressed envelopes might be included to facilitate return of the first-round rating forms, or arrangements may be made to have them sent by overnight courier service. The instructions should remind panellists to review their forms for missing ratings before sending them to the project co-ordinator, and to have a photocopy made of the forms in case they are lost in the mail. Figure 7 shows an example of such a letter, which was sent to panellists who participated in the European panel on the appropriateness of coronary revascularization procedures.

Subject: European Panel on the Appropriateness of Coronary Revascularization Procedures

Dear _____,

Thank you for agreeing to serve on the European panel that will rate the appropriateness of percutaneous transluminal coronary angioplasty (PTCA) and coronary artery bypass graft surgery (CABG) for several European countries. As previously advised, this panel is being carried out under the auspices of the European Commission BIOMED Concerted Action on the appropriateness and necessity of medical and surgical procedures, led by Dr. James Kahan of RAND Europe in Leiden, The Netherlands.

We are pleased to enclose herewith the materials you will need for the first round of appropriateness ratings:

- Coronary Artery Bypass Graft Surgery, Percutaneous Transluminal Coronary Angioplasty or Medical Therapy in Anginal Pain: A Literature Review for Rating Indications (prepared by the Swedish Council on Technology Assessment in Health Care—SBU).
- List of indications to be rated
- Definitions of terms used in the list of indications
- Instructions for rating the list of indications
- Mailing instructions

We are asking you to fill out the rating forms and return them within 2 weeks, that is, no later than Friday, 6 November. Please make a photocopy of your completed rating forms before mailing, so we will have a backup copy in case something gets lost in the mail. The original forms should be sent to us by courier service, as noted in the mailing instructions.

In a few days, we will be calling each of you to confirm that you have received these materials and to discuss any questions or comments you may have about the rating process.

There is no need to bring any materials to Madrid, but you may find it useful to bring the literature review or the definitions, especially if you have made any notes on these documents. At the panel meeting in Madrid, on 18-19 December, you will receive a new set of forms showing how you personally and the panel as a group rated each indication. After discussion of each chapter, led by an experienced panel moderator, panellists will be asked to rate each indication once again.

Should you have any questions, we may be reached at the numbers listed below. Thank you for your participation, and we look forward to welcoming you to Madrid.

Yours sincerely,

Figure 7. Sample Letter to Panellists

Follow-up by phone is important to ensure that everyone has received all the documents and that they understand what is expected of them. This is also a good time to ask the panellists if they have any questions about the indications structure or the definitions. If, as frequently occurs, the panellists have not yet had a chance to review the documents, a specific time should be planned for a return phone call to discuss these issues. These contacts may be made by the panel moderator or someone on the research team, as agreed. Further phone contacts may be necessary to remind panellists of the deadline for returning their ratings or to request their ratings for skipped indications. If more than one or two indications have been missed, however, it is usually easier to fax the pages with the missing ratings to the panellist rather than try to elicit the missing ratings by phone.

The return of the rating forms should be acknowledged, and a reminder given of the date set for the panel meeting. Panellists also need to know whether they are expected to make (and pay for) their own travel arrangements, to be reimbursed subsequently, or if these arrangements can be made for them. If they will be travelling to a foreign city, they might also appreciate knowing what the approximate taxi fare is to the designated hotel.

A letter of welcome should await the panellists on their arrival at the hotel, reminding them when the meeting starts the next morning and how to get to the meeting site. An agenda for the meeting might also be included. If a dinner has been arranged for the group on the night of their arrival—a highly recommended way to give the panellists a chance to become acquainted in an informal setting— the letter should include instructions on when and where to meet.

A few days after the meeting, a personal letter should be sent to each panellist, thanking them for contributing their time and expertise to the project. It is also important to assure that panellists receive a copy of the final product: the appropriateness criteria. If further studies are done, for example, to measure appropriateness in actual patients who have received the procedure, those who have participated on the panel should be informed of the results. Finally, all documents and articles related with the project should acknowledge the panel members by name. Figure 8 shows a checklist for contacts with panellists.

Letter to specialist societies requesting names of candidates. Enclosures: Description of RAND/UCLA appropriateness method in general; description of specific research project (who, what, when, why...).
Informal telephone interviews with selected candidates to explore their interest and availability. Request copy of curriculum vitae from potential candidates.
Letter to candidates inviting participation and suggesting dates Enclosures: Description of RAND/UCLA appropriateness method in general; description of specific research project (who, what, when, why...); explanation of what is expected from them and time commitments involved; form to confirm personal participation and dates available for meeting.
Letter to panellists confirming participation and dates for meeting.
Letter to panellists with documents needed for first round ratings. Enclosures: Literature review; List of indications; Definitions; Instructions for rating, Instructions for returning documents.
Telephone follow-up to confirm receipt of documents, answer questions, explore possible problems with list of indications or definitions.
Phone/fax to panellists to provide missing ratings.
Letter of thanks to panellists for returning first round ratings; Reminder of dates for meeting and instructions on making travel arrangements.
Letter of welcome to panellists when they arrive at the hotel; Instructions on how to get to the meeting site.
Letter of thanks to panellists for their participation in the project
Letter to panellists enclosing final appropriateness criteria.

Figure 8. Checklist for Panellist Contacts

CHAPTER 6. THE RATING PROCESS: APPROPRIATENESS AND NECESSITY

Introduction

The development of appropriateness criteria usually involves two rounds of rating: panellists are asked to rate the list of indications first, independently, in their home or place of work, and second, during a structured meeting led by an experienced moderator, at which all panellists are present. In each case, they are asked to rate the appropriateness of performing a procedure (or providing a treatment) for each clinical scenario by circling a number from 1 to 9, where 1 indicates that it is highly inappropriate and 9 that it is highly appropriate. A procedure or treatment is considered to be appropriate if:

> "The expected health benefit (e.g., increased life expectancy, relief
> of pain, reduction in anxiety, improved functional capacity)
> exceeds the expected negative consequences (e.g., mortality,
> morbidity, anxiety, pain, time lost from work) by a sufficiently
> wide margin that the procedure is worth doing, exclusive of cost."
> (Brook et al., 1986)

Panellists are asked to rate the appropriateness of each indication using their own best clinical judgement (rather than their perceptions of what other experts might say) and considering an average patient presenting to an average physician who performs the procedure in an average hospital (or other care-providing facility). *They are specifically instructed **not** to consider cost implications in making their judgements.* Although cost considerations are an important factor in deciding whether a procedure or treatment should ultimately be made available to patients, the RAM focuses on the initial question of whether it is effective. Once physicians judge a treatment or procedure as effective, then a broader group of individuals—consumers, patients and payers—should also be included in the discussion.

The development of necessity criteria involves a third (and sometimes a fourth) round of ratings, usually by mail, in which panellists rate only the subset of indications that were judged appropriate by the panel in the second round. A procedure is considered *necessary* when *all* of the following criteria are met:

- The procedure must be appropriate (that is, it must have a median rating of 7, 8 or 9 without disagreement on the final appropriateness scale).
- It would be considered improper care not to provide this service.
- There is a reasonable chance that this procedure will benefit the patient. (A procedure could be appropriate if it had a low likelihood of benefit but few risks; such procedures would not be necessary.)
- The benefit to the patient is not small. (A procedure could be appropriate if it had a minor but almost certain benefit, but it would not be necessary.)

Necessity is thus a more stringent criterion than appropriateness. If a procedure is necessary, this means not only that the expected benefits outweigh the expected harms (i.e., it is appropriate), but that they do so by such a margin that the physician *must* offer the service. One might say that "the care is so clearly the right thing to do that the physician would believe it unethical not to provide it and might anticipate being sued...if he or she did not offer it to the patient" (Brook, 1999). Of course, patients may decline to follow their physician's recommendations.

Panellists rate necessity using a 1 to 9 scale similar to that used for rating appropriateness. A high rating on this scale means that it is improper clinical judgement not to recommend the procedure. A low rating means that, although the procedure is appropriate, it is not necessary.

Rating Appropriateness: First Round

For the first-round ratings panellists receive by mail, along with the rating forms, the following documents: the literature review, list of indications, definitions of terms, and instructions for rating. It is important to give them specific instructions about when the completed list should be returned (4-6 weeks should be sufficient), how it should be returned (by courier service if the project can afford to pay the cost), and whom to call if they need help (phone, fax and email address should be provided). At this point in the process, panellists usually do not know the identity of the other members of the panel (unless a round zero meeting was previously held, as discussed in Chapter 4).

The instructions given to panellists should explain that the purpose of the literature review is to provide them with an up-to-date summary of the scientific evidence regarding the procedure in question. Depending on the length and complexity of this document, they might expect to spend 5-10 hours reading it. The instructions should also emphasise the importance of taking the time to study the structure of the list of indications before rating the indications. The experience of panellists in previous studies has shown that filling in the first few pages takes the most time and may cause the most frustration. It may also help to suggest that the panellists begin by rating a chapter that has a relatively simple structure, not necessarily the first chapter. Once they understand the logic of the structure, the rating will go much faster. Panellists should circle their ratings in pencil, in case they want to go back and change any of them later. On average, about 150-200 indications can be rated in an hour once the panellist is used to the process.

After the panellists have received their documents, the panel moderator, or a member of the research group, should contact each one by phone to assure that they understand the process and to explore possible problems with either the structure of the list of indications or the definitions of the terms used in the list. Panellists should be forewarned that they will be receiving a call, so that they are prepared to respond. The moderator should make a note of all comments received, so that these can be discussed at the panel meeting. If major changes to the structure of the list of indications are suggested, it may be necessary to prepare new forms for whatever chapters are affected. A decision to collapse categories can easily be handled during the second-round ratings, as can a decision to add one new category or change the boundaries of existing categories. Anything more sophisticated than these types of changes, however, will probably require the preparation of new forms.

Panellists who have not returned their forms by the last week of the designated period should be contacted to find out when they anticipate completing them. A certain margin should be built into the calendar to allow for the fact that a few panellists will always return their forms late. They should be asked to review their forms for "missing" ratings before sending them, and to make a photocopy of the forms in case something gets lost in the mail. Inevitably, however, there will be missing data as it is very difficult to rate hundreds or possibly thousands of indications without skipping at least a few of them. Sheets with missing ratings can be faxed to the panellists with an indication of which ones need to be filled in. Figure 9 shows an example of a completed first-round rating sheet from the European panel on coronary revascularization.[1]

Each panellist should be assigned a number, which is used to identify their rating forms (panellist number 1, panellist number 2, and so on). At the panel meeting, name-cards can be placed at the table in this same order to help the panel moderator identify each person.

As the first round forms are received, the research team will enter the ratings in a database so that the second round forms can be produced. It is strongly recommended that data be entered twice, in two separate databases, so that any data entry errors will be caught when comparing the two. Alternatively, if the research team has access to and experience with optical scanning devices, these might also be used.

Rating Appropriateness: Second Round

The second round of ratings is done during the panel meeting. Here, panellists will receive a set of forms similar to the ones they used to rate in the first round, but with additional information about how the panel as a whole and they as individuals rated each indication. These second round forms show the frequency of responses for each indication, as well as the individual panellist's own response. This document forms the basis for the discussion during the panel meeting.

The purpose of the second round is to give the panellists the opportunity to discuss their ratings face to face, in light of their knowledge of how all the other panellists rated. Generally, the panel moderator will focus on indications where there is considerable dispersion in the panel ratings to find out if there is genuine clinical disagreement about appropriateness or if there is a problem with the rating structure. Each chapter is discussed in detail, after which the panellists are asked to re-rate all the indications in the chapter (or section, if the chapters are very long), regardless of whether their ratings are unchanged from the first round. After each chapter is re-rated (which may take from 10 minutes to half an

---

[1] It will be noted that, in addition to rating the appropriateness of PTCA and CABG for each indication, this particular panel also rated the perceived quality of the evidence on which their decision was based.

Round 1. Panelist 8

CHAPTER 2

UNSTABLE ANGINA

	LOW/MODERATE Surgical Risk						HIGH Surgical Risk						
	PTCA		CABG			PTCA		CABG			(Indic. No.)

C. PATIENT HAS NO SYMPTOMS (NOT ON IV NITRATES)

1. Left main disease

2. Three vessel disease

a) With very positive stress test

1) LVEF >=50%

2) LVEF >=30% - <50%

3) LVEF >=20% - <30%

b) With moderately positive stress test

1) LVEF >=50%

2) LVEF >=30% - <50%

3) LVEF >=20% - <30%

c) With stress test indeterminate or not done

1) LVEF >=50%

2) LVEF >=30% - <50%

3) LVEF >=20% - <30%

d) With negative stress test

1) LVEF >=50%

2) LVEF >=30% - <50%

3) LVEF >=20% - <30%

APPROPRIATENESS SCALE:
1 = Extremely inappropriate
9 = Extremely appropriate

EVIDENCE SCALE:
A = Convincing scientific evidence
B = Weaker scientific evidence
C = Expert opinion
D = Your own experience/opinion or that of your peers

Figure 9. Sample First Round Rating Sheet, European Panel on Coronary Revascularization, December 1998

hour depending on its length), the forms should immediately be checked for completeness. Panellists should be asked to fill in any missing ratings before moving on to the discussion of the next chapter. It is a good idea to offer panellists frequent breaks, for example, after they re-rate each chapter, to avoid over-tiring them. Drinks and light snacks should be made available at some of these breaks, or they may be placed on a table in the meeting room so that they are available throughout the meeting.

Documents Required

Appropriateness panels require the preparation of various kinds of forms for use of the panellists and the moderator. An example of a first round rating sheet was shown in Figure 9 of this chapter. For the second round—the panel meeting—a customised set of forms is prepared for each panellist, showing how the panel as a group rated each indication, together with the panellist's own response. Two sets of forms are usually prepared for the moderator, one showing the group rating, the level of agreement and the level of appropriateness with which each indication was rated (and sometimes additional information), and the other showing the individual rating of each panellist for each indication. These documents are discussed in more detail below.

Personalised Panellist Rating Sheet

This document is unique for each panellist. It shows the frequency of responses for each indication, together with a symbol indicating the panellist's own response, typically in the following format:

Indication xxxxxxxx	8 3 2 1 1 1 2 3 4 5 6 7 8 9

In the preceding example, eight panellists rated the indication a 1 (highly inappropriate), three panellists rated it a 2, two panellists rated it a 3, one panellist rated it a 5, and one panellist rated it a 6. This particular panellist rated it a 1.

Depending on the software used to produce the forms, other options would be to put a caret (^) under the panellist's rating, or to put an asterisk (*) beside or in replacement of the panellist's own response, as shown in the following examples:

```
                          6 2 2 1 2 1        1
   Indication xxxxxxx      1 2 3 4 5 6 7 8 9    (2.0, 1.8)
                           ^
```

```
                          6 2 2 1 2 1        1
   Indication xxxxxxx      1*2 3 4 5 6 7 8 9    (2.0, 1.8)
```

```
                          6 2 2 1 2 1         1
   Indication xxxxxxx      * 2 3 4 5 6 7 8 9    (2.0, 1.8)
```

Sometimes the median and a statistic indicating the dispersion of the ratings (for example, the mean absolute deviation from the median) are also included, as shown above. In these examples, six panellists rated a 1, two panellists rated a 2, two panellists rated a 3, and so on. This particular panellist rated a 1. The median rating was 2 and the mean absolute deviation from the median was 1.8. It can be helpful to use a different type style and/or size for the frequency of responses so they are not confused with the numbers in the scale.

An example of a personalised rating sheet used in the second round ratings is shown in Figure 10. It shows the same page from the panellist whose first round sheet is shown in Figure 9. Note the heading indicating that this form is for panellist number 8. It is important to assure that each panellist receives the correct set of forms, in accordance with the panellist number previously assigned. The last column in this form shows the indication numbers for the indications contained in each row.

If we compare the first indication shown in each figure (indication number 341), it can be seen that this panellist rated a 1 on the appropriateness scale for PTCA in the first round, and this is reflected in the second round sheet by putting an asterisk after that rating (1*). The second round ratings are entered directly on the personalised ratings sheets. Panellists are asked to re-rate each indication by circling a number on the appropriateness scale, even when they wish to rate the indication exactly the same as they did in the first round.

Round 2, Panelist 8

CHAPTER 2	LOW/MODERATE Surgical Risk		HIGH Surgical Risk		Indic. No.
UNSTABLE ANGINA	PTCA	CABG	CABG	PTCA	
	Appropriateness — Evidence	Appropriateness — Evidence	Appropriateness — Evidence	Appropriateness — Evidence	

C. PATIENT HAS NO SYMPTOMS (NOT ON IV NITRATES)

1. Left main disease — 341-344

2. Three vessel disease

a) With very positive stress test

1) EF >=50% — 345-348
2) EF >=30-<50% — 349-352
3) EF >=20-<30% — 353-356

b) With moderately positive stress test

1) EF >=50% — 357-360
2) EF >=30-<50% — 361-364
3) EF >=20-<30% — 365-368

c) With stress test indeterminate or not done

1) EF >=50% — 369-372
2) EF >=30-<50% — 373-376
3) EF >=20-<30% — 377-380

d) With negative stress test

1) EF >=50% — 381-384
2) EF >=30-<50% — 385-388
3) EF >=20-<30% — 389-392

APPROPRIATENESS SCALE: 1 = Extremely inappropriate   9 = Extremely appropriate

EVIDENCE SCALE:
A = Convincing scientific evidence
B = Weaker scientific evidence
C = Expert opinion
D = Your own experience/opinion or that of your peers

Figure 10. Sample Second Round Rating Sheet, European Panel on Coronary Revascularization, December 1998

Moderator's Summary Rating Form

The moderator works with two documents to prepare and carry out the panel meeting. The summary rating form, like the personalised panellist document, shows the frequency of responses for each indication. In addition, this document includes other information that helps the moderator decide which indications to highlight for discussion during the meeting: the median (and sometimes a measure of dispersion), the level of agreement with which the indication was rated (agreement, indeterminate, disagreement), and the appropriateness rating (appropriate, uncertain, inappropriate). The latter two variables can be shown in different ways, for example, using letters and/or symbols, as follows:

							1	*1*		*6*	*2*	*5*			
Indication xxxxxxxxx	1	2	3	4	5	6	7	8	9				**7 A +**		

In this example, 7 is the median rating, A means the indication is appropriate (U would be uncertain and I inappropriate), and + means that it was rated with agreement (? would be indeterminate and—would be disagreement). Other ways of displaying information have been used, including manually colour-highlighting the indications for which disagreement exists. This form is often used extensively by the moderator during the panel meeting to help identify indications to be discussed. See Chapter 7 for more information on how the moderator uses this document to guide the discussion.

Moderator's Detailed Panellist Rating Form

The detailed panellist rating form shows how each individual panellist rated each indication. It is generally used more in preparing for the meeting than during the meeting itself. In this document the numbers on the bottom line do not represent the appropriateness scale, but rather individual panellists, as shown in the following example:

	9	**8**	**2**	**9**	**9**	**7**	**6**	**8**	**5**	**9**	**8**	**7**	
Indication xxxxxxxxx	1	2	3	4	5	6	7	8	9	10	11	12	**8 A +**

In the above example, there are 12 panellists. Panellist number one rated a 9, panellist number two rated an 8, panellist number three rated a 2, and so on. The main use for this document is to identify panellists who rate very differently from the rest of the panel. The moderator might use this information to try to find out during the discussion why a particular panellist had divergent ratings.

Automating the Rating Process

Some panels have experimented with the use of machine-readable (i.e., optical scanner) forms for panellist ratings. These experiences have shown that, with the technology available at the time, this process was not cost-effective. Some users of the appropriateness method have also raised the idea of having the panellists input their ratings directly on personal computers. Although this is technically feasible, the experimental computer programs that have been written to explore this possibility suffer from a major limitation: they allow the panellist to look at just one screenful of data at a time, whereas experience has shown that panellists like to flip back and forth between pages to compare their ratings. This can be done much more easily in paper than in electronic format, and the ability to do so is likely to improve intra-panellist consistency. Another argument against automating the rating process is that panellists often like to do the ratings during business travel or while on vacation, times at which it may not be convenient or possible to take along a computer. Further investigations are being made into the possibility of using "group decision rooms" where all panellists are provided with a means for direct on-line rating in addition to both face-to-face and written discussion. In such an environment, more rapid rating and better understanding of the reasoning behind the ratings may be possible.

Other Materials and Resources for the Panel Meeting

In addition to the documents described, each panellist should also be provided with a copy of the definitions of the terms used in the list of indications, as it is often necessary to refer to this document during the discussion. Several copies of the literature review should also be on hand in case someone wants to refer to a specific study mentioned in the review. It may also be helpful to have copies of important articles available at the meeting.

Name-cards should be placed on the table before the meeting to assure that panellists sit in the order of their assigned numbers (panellist 1, panellist 2, etc.)

and that they have the correct personalised rating forms. This will also help the panellists and moderator recognise each other by name from the outset. Providing notepads and pens or pencils is also a good idea.

At least two or three support staff members should be on hand during the panel meeting to handle paperwork and logistics. These persons will be needed to help check over the rating forms for completeness, to make photocopies if necessary, and to assist panellists with travel or other matters. Depending on the moderator's clinical knowledge, it may also help to have a "content expert" at the meeting, for example, a member of the study team with in-depth knowledge of the topic, such as the person who conducted the literature review. If the panellists are asked to rate necessity during the panel meeting, data entry staff will also need to be on hand to produce the new forms on very short notice.

One member of the research team should be assigned to take notes during the panel discussion so that the most important issues covered are well documented (for example, revised definitions, changes in the wording of indications). Some panels have experimented with audio or video-taping the entire proceedings, but transcribing the results in a useful format can be difficult and expensive, so this is not frequently done.

It has become common practice to ask the panellists to fill out a "post-panel questionnaire, " which gives them an opportunity to comment on the entire rating process and their experience of the panel meeting. An example of one frequently used form is shown in Figure 11.

Finally, it will be easier for panellists to mail in their requests for reimbursement after the panel meeting if they are provided with a form reminding them to supply relevant bank information and to attach supporting receipts. The name and mailing address of the person responsible for processing this information should be clearly marked on the form.

Thank you for participating in our study of _____. As a final favour, we would appreciate your completing this questionnaire about your experience as a participant. For each item, please circle the appropriate number or fill in the blank. If you have any additional comments or suggestions, please note them on the attached page.

Item	Not at all	A little	Some-what	Pretty much	Very much
	1	2	3	4	5
REVIEW OF THE SCIENTIFIC LITERATURE					
How completely did you read it?	1	2	3	4	5
How many hours did you spend reading it?	___ hrs.				
How objective was it?	1	2	3	4	5
How informative was it?	1	2	3	4	5
How much did it influence your first round ratings?	1	2	3	4	5
FIRST ROUND RATINGS (done before the meeting)					
How easy did you find the task?	1	2	3	4	5
How onerous did you find the task?	1	2	3	4	5
How clear were the instructions?	1	2	3	4	5
How inconsistent do you believe you were? (due to effects of fatigue, memory, different times to rate, format of instrument, etc.)	1	2	3	4	5
How many hours did it take you to complete all the ratings?	___ hrs.				
PANEL MEETING					
How well did the moderator function as a group leader?	1	2	3	4	5
How informative was the discussion?	1	2	3	4	5
How argumentative was the discussion?	1	2	3	4	5
How much did the feedback from the first round ratings influence your second round ratings?	1	2	3	4	5
How much did the discussion influence your second round ratings?	1	2	3	4	5
OVERALL IMPRESSIONS OF YOUR EXPERIENCE					
How well do you believe *your own* ratings reflect the appropriateness of revascularization procedures?	1	2	3	4	5
How well do you believe *the panel's* ratings will reflect the appropriateness of revascularization procedures?	1	2	3	4	5
How much do you believe that this panel process can lead to a set of recommendations to assist physician decision-making for revascularization?	1	2	3	4	5
How satisfying did you find your participation on this panel?	1	2	3	4	5
How did your participation on this panel compare with your expectations?	much worse	worse	on a par	better	much better

Figure 11. Sample Post-Panel Questionnaire

Figure 12 shows a checklist of suggested materials that should be available during the meeting at which the second round ratings take place.

For Panellists:

- Personalised panellist rating sheets (frequencies; own ratings)
- Definitions
- Literature review
- Pencils, erasers, pencil sharpeners
- Name cards on table (in same order as seating chart)
- Agenda for meeting (indicating coffee breaks, lunch)
- List of panel members and observers, with their affiliations
- Post-panel questionnaire
- Reimbursement form

For Moderator:

- Moderator summary rating form (frequencies; median; classification of appropriateness and agreement)
- Moderator detailed panellist rating form (individual panellist ratings)
- Seating chart
- Overhead (or slide) projector and screen
- Flipchart and coloured markers (or blackboard and chalk)

Figure 12. Checklist of Materials for Second Round Ratings

Panel Observers

Most appropriateness panel meetings include a number of silent observers. These may be persons who have worked on the literature review or the list of indications, persons who are interested in applying the appropriateness method to a procedure of their own interest, or perhaps potential panel moderators who would like to see an experienced moderator in action. Whatever their interest, they should at all times respect the work of the panel by remaining silent and not creating distractions or interruptions. The observers should sit around the sides of the room, never at the same table with the panellists. All such observers should be introduced to the panel at the beginning of the meeting or shortly after they enter the room. Past experience has shown that the presence of a small "audience" of this type has no negative effect on the panel process.

A specialist in the subject matter or an expert in applying the methodology may also be among the observers; these persons may, on rare occasion, wish to speak from the sideline, but they should refrain from making long speeches and should be careful never to argue in public with the moderator. Occasionally, this specialist may be seated at the table to provide "content advice" to the moderator.

Rating Necessity: Third Round

If a rating of necessity is to take place after the two ratings of appropriateness, panellists should be informed of this at the end of the panel meeting. The moderator will want to explain the difference between appropriateness and necessity, clearly specifying that "not necessary" means only that the procedure does not *have to* be done, not that it *should* not be done. Thus, in the final classification each indication would be labelled as either:

- Appropriate and necessary
- Appropriate but not necessary
- Uncertain
- Inappropriate

Panellists need to understand the purpose of developing necessity criteria— that they may be used to detect underuse by determining which patients who might have benefited from the procedure did not receive it. For example, studies have been done of patients who have undergone coronary angiography to determine what proportion of those meeting the criteria for a necessary revascularization procedure actually received it (Kravitz et al., 1995).

The list of indications to be rated for necessity includes only those indications that were classified as appropriate by the panel in the second round ratings, that is, all indications for which the median panel rating was between 7 and 9, without disagreement. A sample form for rating necessity, taken from the European panel on gastrointestinal endoscopy, is shown in Figure 13. As can be seen, the original indications matrix is maintained, but the 1-9 scale is replaced by a dotted line for those indications that are not to be rated for necessity (because they were not classified as "appropriate" in the second-round ratings). The forms for rating necessity are usually sent to the panellists by mail, although if panellist time and project resources permit, it is also possible to rate necessity during the panel meeting. For example, the European endoscopy panel appropriateness ratings were processed overnight following the first day of the meeting so that necessity could be rated the morning of the second day. This required the availability of computers and trained personnel on site to enter the data and quickly prepare the new forms. Alternatively, a Swedish coronary revascularization panel rated necessity in two rounds, first, by mail, and second, after group discussion, similar to the two-round process used in rating appropriateness (Johansson et al., 1994).

If the necessity ratings are done by mail, it is a good idea to send the new forms within a month of the panel meeting, while the rating process is still fresh in the panellists' minds. Clear instructions should be included, reminding the panel of the definition of necessity and the reason for producing these criteria. Just as in the first round, a reasonable deadline should be set for return of the forms—perhaps 2 to 4 weeks, depending on the length of the indications list. Experience has shown that frequent follow-ups are often needed to assure that all panellists return the completed forms.

CHAPTER 1
Upper Gastro-Intestinal Endoscopy for Uncomplicated Dyspepsia
A. No previous investigation or results unknown (cont.)

	Less than 45 years old		45 years or older		Indication number
	NSAID	No NSAID	NSAID	No NSAID	
4. HP test negative, empiric acid lowering treatment given					
a) Symptoms resolved	....	....	....	....	(25-28)
b) Symptoms not resolved	....	....	1 2 3 4 5 6 7 8 9	1 2 3 4 5 6 7 8 9	(29-32)
5. HP test positive, no HP eradication treatment					
a) Symptoms resolved	....	....	....	....	(33-36)
b) Symptoms not resolved	....	....	1 2 3 4 5 6 7 8 9	1 2 3 4 5 6 7 8 9	(37-40)
6. HP test positive, HP eradication treatment given					
a) Symptoms resolved	....	....	....	....	(41-44)
b) Symptoms not resolved	1 2 3 4 5 6 7 8 9	1 2 3 4 5 6 7 8 9	1 2 3 4 5 6 7 8 9	1 2 3 4 5 6 7 8 9	(45-48)

Necessity scale: 1 = clearly not necessary, 5 = might be necessary, 9 = clearly necessary.

Figure 13. Sample Form for Rating Necessity, European Gastrointestinal Endoscopy Panel, November 1998

CHAPTER 7. CHAIRING AN EXPERT PANEL

The Moderator

The most important individual in the panel process is the panel moderator. This person is generally a physician, but preferably not a specialist in the procedure being rated, in order to avoid bringing his or her own biases to the discussion. The moderator must know how to deal with panellists, and should have a broad understanding of both the topics to be discussed and the outcomes needed from the panel process. At an absolute minimum, the moderator should be very familiar with the literature review and comfortable with the material. Ideally, the moderator should also assist in the literature review (see Chapter 3). Of course, the moderator must also be fluent in the language(s) in which the panel will be conducted. Sometimes two moderators are used: one a physician, and the other a person more experienced in applying the RAM. Highly recommended—and the best possible preparation for conducting a RAM expert panel meeting—is the opportunity to observe an experienced moderator in action.

Preparing for the Meeting

The panel moderator should contact each panellist between the first and second rounds of ratings to discuss any concerns they may have and to let the panellists know they are making a significant contribution to the process. It is particularly important to find out if the panellists believe the structure of the list of indications adequately reflects the full range of patients who might present for the procedure under study. They should also be reminded to review the definitions provided for the terms used in the list of indications to see if they have any modifications to suggest.

Once the first round results have been tabulated and the moderator forms produced, these should be carefully reviewed to identify areas to be discussed during the panel meeting. Depending on the moderator's previous experience with the RAM, this will require between one and two days of preparation. One way to review the first round ratings in a structured manner is to colour code the rating sheets. There are no hard and fast rules for doing this; rather, the choice of which indications to highlight depends on what the moderator wants the panel to focus on. One experienced moderator uses a code based on traffic lights: indications that are appropriate are highlighted in green, those that are inappropriate are highlighted in pink, and those that are uncertain are highlighted in yellow. It will be recalled that indications may be uncertain either because: 1) most panellists rate them toward the middle of the scale; 2) the panellists are widely polarised in their ratings; or 3) the panellists' ratings are scattered along the entire scale. Any of these distributions will yield a median in the middle of the scale. Another approach might be to highlight indications that are rated with agreement in green, those that are rated with disagreement in pink, and those that are considered indeterminate with respect to agreement (i.e., neither agreement nor disagreement) are highlighted in yellow or left without colour. Figure 14 shows an example of how a moderator might highlight the indications to be discussed during the meeting based on the panel's level of agreement. In this example, the light shading represents agreement, the dark shading represents disagreement and those indications without shading were indeterminate with respect to agreement. In this figure, it will also be noticed that the panel's median rating is shown numerically to the right of each indication, as are symbols the representing level of agreement (+, -, ?) and the appropriateness of the indication (Appropriate, Uncertain, Disagreement).

The main purpose of this methodical review is to identify 1) indications that have been rated with disagreement and 2) inconsistencies in appropriateness ratings. For example, in a coronary revascularization panel it might be noted that, for a certain group of indications, some panellists tend to rate at one end of the scale while others tend to rate at the other (producing disagreement). Why does this occur? It may be that some panellists are thinking of one set of patients while others are thinking of another, suggesting an indication that is not homogeneous and needs to be specified in more detail. More concretely, if "mild angina" is defined to include class I and class II angina, and panellists think differently about patients in these two categories, it may be necessary to re-rate the indications in the second round, first for class I angina and again for class II angina. (See "Modifying the Indications Matrix during the Panel Meeting," in this chapter, for how this can be done).

CHAPTER 1
CHRONIC STABLE ANGINA

	LOW/MODERATE Surgical Risk		HIGH Surgical Risk		Indic No.
	PTCA Appropriateness	CABG Appropriateness	PTCA Appropriateness	CABG Appropriateness	

SEVERE ANGINA (CLASS III/IV)

4. One or two vessel without PLAD

a) Very positive stress test

	PTCA (LOW/MOD)	CABG (LOW/MOD)	PTCA (HIGH)	CABG (HIGH)	Indic No.
EF>=50	1 4 1 9 · 1 2 3 4 5 6 7 8 9 · 9 +A	3 2 1 1 3 2 3 · 1 2 3 4 5 6 7 8 9 · 7 - U	4 2 9 · 1 2 3 4 5 6 7 8 9 · 9 +A	3 2 2 1 2 2 2 1 5 · 1 2 3 4 5 6 7 8 9 · - U	65-68
EF30-<50	1 3 3 8 · 1 2 3 4 5 6 7 8 9 · 9 +A	1 2 1 2 4 2 3 · 1 2 3 4 5 6 7 8 9 · 7 ? A	3 4 8 · 1 2 3 4 5 6 7 8 9 · 9 +A	1 3 2 1 3 2 2 1 6 · 1 2 3 4 5 6 7 8 9 · ? U	69-72
EF20-<30	2 5 3 5 · 1 2 3 4 5 6 7 8 9 · 8 +A	1 1 1 3 1 4 · 1 2 3 4 5 6 7 8 9 · 7 ? A	1 5 4 5 · 1 2 3 4 5 6 7 8 9 · 8 +A	1 2 1 2 1 3 2 2 1 6 · 1 2 3 4 5 6 7 8 9 · ? U	73-76

b) Moderately positive stress test

	PTCA (LOW/MOD)	CABG (LOW/MOD)	PTCA (HIGH)	CABG (HIGH)	Indic No.
EF>=50	1 4 2 8 · 1 2 3 4 5 6 7 8 9 · 9 +A	1 2 2 1 1 2 3 2 6 · 1 2 3 4 5 6 7 8 9 · - U	1 5 2 7 · 1 2 3 4 5 6 7 8 9 · 8 +A	3 2 1 1 3 2 1 1 5 · 1 2 3 4 5 6 7 8 9 · - U	77-80
EF30-<50	1 3 5 6 · 1 2 3 4 5 6 7 8 9 · 8 +A	1 2 2 2 3 3 2 7 · 1 2 3 4 5 6 7 8 9 · ? A	1 4 4 6 · 1 2 3 4 5 6 7 8 9 · 8 +A	1 3 1 1 1 4 1 2 1 6 · 1 2 3 4 5 6 7 8 9 · ? U	81-84
EF20-<30	1 1 6 4 3 · 1 2 3 4 5 6 7 8 9 · 7 +A	1 1 2 3 1 3 1 3 6 · 1 2 3 4 5 6 7 8 9 · ? U	1 1 6 4 3 · 1 2 3 4 5 6 7 8 9 · 7 +A	1 2 2 1 1 4 1 2 1 6 · 1 2 3 4 5 6 7 8 9 · ? U	85-88

A = Appropriate
U = Uncertain
I = Inappropriate

= agreement (+)
= disagreement (-)
= indeterminate (?)

Figure 14. Sample Colour-Coded Moderator Sheet from a 15 Member European Coronary Revascularization Panel

Continuing the example of a coronary revascularization panel, identification of which panellists rated in each extreme (using the moderator's detailed panellist rating form discussed in Chapter 6) might show that the cardiologists tended to think that angioplasty was highly appropriate for this particular indication, while the cardiovascular surgeons tended to think it was highly inappropriate. Thus, disagreement may represent genuine differences of clinical opinion held by each speciality group (or by individuals). It is the job of the moderator to detect these kinds of differences so they can be discussed during the meeting.

The second—and more difficult—task of the moderator in reviewing the first round ratings is to highlight inconsistencies in the appropriateness ratings. For example, it may be noted that, for most indications, coronary revascularization is considered progressively more appropriate with decreasing ejection fraction. But there may be some instances in which, according to the panel ratings, it is uncertain when the patient's ejection fraction is high, appropriate when it is intermediate, and uncertain when it is low. The moderator may want to call the panel's attention to such apparent discrepancies during the meeting so they can discuss if there is a clinical basis for them. These types of pattern inconsistencies can also be identified by computer programs (Kravitz et al, 1997; McDonnell et al., 1996).

The moderator may also notice in reviewing the first round ratings that some variables do not appear to influence the panellists' thinking and might be eliminated. For example, if appropriateness ratings are always the same for patients under 65 and over 65, it may not be necessary to include age group as a separate variable. Thus, the matrix can be collapsed, reducing the number of indications to be re-rated.

Alternatively, the panellists may consider that age 75 rather than 65 is a better threshold for where their decisions would differ. One method to automatically identify appropriate cut-off points is the use of a computerised classification and regression tree (CART) program. However, these programs must be used carefully so their results make clinical sense.

At the Meeting

At the beginning of the panel meeting it is important to review the purpose of the study. Examples can be given of the wide clinical practice variations that have been documented in different geographic regions and the potential over- or underuse of medical procedures. The panel moderator should emphasise that the study is designed to determine the best care for individual patients, and that it is not solely an academic exercise. Panellists will want to know how their ratings will be used. For example, the appropriateness ratings might be applied to clinical records to measure appropriateness retrospectively, or they could be used as a basis for forming a set of clinical recommendations or other aids to clinical decision-making. It is important for the panel to understand that the method is not necessarily an attempt to reduce the number of procedures being done or to control costs, as both underuse and overuse of the same procedure may very well occur at the same time. Rather, the focus is on assuring that the procedure in question is selectively used only in patients who are truly likely to benefit from it. Where the results of the panel indicate uncertainty as to the appropriateness of the procedure, this can help determine where properly designed randomised controlled trials might be of most value.

Before beginning the panel discussion, it is also worthwhile to take the time to explain the appropriateness methodology so that all panellists understand what is expected of them. The moderator should also carefully review the format of the rating forms and note that each indication is numbered for entry identification (see the last column in Figure 14, labelled "Indic. No."). It is particularly important to emphasise that the purpose of the meeting is not to force the panel to consensus. Brief mention might be made of other types of so-called "consensus methods" in which panellists *are* expected to agree on their conclusions, stressing that the appropriateness method specifically does *not* have this objective. It should also be noted that cost considerations—while they might well come into play at a policy making level later on—should not be considered in rating appropriateness. Finally, panellists should be encouraged to use the full scale for their ratings, and to base their ratings, insofar as possible, on the available scientific evidence rather than personal opinion. For example, in order to emphasise the type and quality of available evidence, the investigators of the European endoscopy panel presented a brief oral summary of existing evidence to the panellists before each chapter was discussed and re-rated.

Following this introduction to the method and discussion of any questions the panellists might have, the moderator will begin the discussion, usually with the first chapter in the list of indications. Alternatively, if the first chapter is quite long and/or complicated, the moderator might decide to begin the discussion with a chapter that is shorter and easier, even if it is not the first one presented in the rating booklet. This will help panellists to familiarise themselves with the process without having to try to understand a very complex chapter. In either case, the initial chapter invariably takes longer (sometimes much longer) than succeeding chapters, as panellists are "warming up". This should not be a cause for concern.

Modifying the List of Indications (During the Panel Meeting)

The panel discussion may reveal that some of the disagreement in the first-round ratings occurred because panellists are thinking about different patients within the same clinical indication. That is, the indications may not be sufficiently homogeneous. If this occurs, a way must be found to redefine the structure of the list of indications so that such differences can be resolved. This may involve changing the categories for a particular variable, or adding new categories or variables. If the problem is to redefine or eliminate existing categories, panellists can simply note the changes on their rating sheets, as shown in Figure 15. In this case, a panel examining the appropriateness of coronary revascularization decided that there were no significant differences in their ratings between patients with a left ventricular ejection fraction (LVEF) of >20% and ≤30% and those with an LVEF of >30% and ≤50%. Therefore they combined these two categories and created a new category of LVEF >20% and ≤50%.

A) Before the Meeting		B) At the Meeting	
LVEF a) >50%	1 2 3 4 5 6 7 8 9	LVEF a) >50%	1 2 3 4 5 6 7 8 9
b) >30% and ≤50%	1 2 3 4 5 6 7 8 9	b) >20% and ≤50%	1 2 3 4 5 6 7 8 9
c) >20% and ≤30%	1 2 3 4 5 6 7 8 9	~~c) >20% and ≤30%~~	~~1 2 3 4 5 6 7 8 9~~

Figure 15. Eliminating a Category from the List of Indications

If, on the other hand, a new category needs to be added, panellists can use circles (0) and ex's (X) to expand the structure, as seen in Figure 16. In this example, panellists decided they did not want to include patients with negative and inconclusive stress test results in the same category because they thought differently about these two types of patients. Therefore, in part A) below, the circles represent the appropriateness ratings for patients with a negative stress test while the X's represent the ratings for those with an inconclusive test. The moderator should write the definitions of the 0's and X's on the blackboard or a flipchart, and ask panellists to copy them onto their rating sheets, to be sure everyone understands how they are being used. Following the meeting, the indications now appear as shown in part B of Figure 16.

A) At the Meeting	B) Following the Meeting
Two-vessel disease with proximal left anterior descending involvement	Two-vessel disease with proximal left anterior descending involvement
a) Positive stress test	a) Positive stress test
LVEF a) >50%　　1 2 3 4 5 6 7 8 ⑨	LVEF a) >50%　　1 2 3 4 5 6 7 8 ⑨
b) >30% and ≤50%　1 2 3 4 5 6 7 8 ⑨	b) >30% and ≤50%　1 2 3 4 5 6 7 8 ⑨
c) >20% and ≤30%　1 2 3 4 5 6 7 ⑧ 9	c) >20% and ≤30%　1 2 3 4 5 6 7 ⑧ 9
b) Negative or inconclusive stress test	b) Inconclusive stress test
LVEF a) >50%　　1 2 3 4 5 ⑥ ✗ 8 9	LVEF a) >50%　　1 2 3 4 5 6 ⑦ 8 9
b) >30% and ≤50%　1 2 3 4 5 ⑥ ✗ 8 9	b) >30% and ≤50%　1 2 3 4 5 6 ⑦ 8 9
c) >20% and ≤30%　1 2 3 4 5 ⑥ ✗ 8 9	c) >20% and ≤30%　1 2 3 4 5 6 ⑦ 8 9
c) Stress test not done	c) Negative stress test
LVEF a) >50%　　1 2 3 4 5 6 7 ⑧ 9	LVEF a) >50%　　1 2 3 4 5 ⑥ 7 8 9
b) >30% and ≤50%　1 2 3 4 5 6 7 ⑧ 9	b) >30% and ≤50%　1 2 3 4 5 ⑥ 7 8 9
c) >20% and ≤30%　1 2 3 4 5 ⑥ 7 8 9	c) >20% and ≤30%　1 2 3 4 5 ⑥ 7 8 9
	d) Stress test not done
	LVEF a) >50%　　1 2 3 4 5 6 ⑦⑧ 9
◯ = negative	b) >30% and ≤50%　1 2 3 4 5 6 ⑦⑧ 9
✗ = inconclusive	c) >20% and ≤30%　1 2 3 4 5 ⑥ 7 8 9

Figure 16. Adding a Category to the List of Indications

The moderator should not, however, be too quick to suggest that indications be split or joined; rather, sufficient discussion should be encouraged to assure that there is wide agreement among the panel about the need to modify the structure. On occasion, panellists may start out believing that such changes need to be made, only to conclude after further discussion that they would not really affect their appropriateness ratings.

Guiding the Discussion

A good moderator will neither dominate the discussion nor let the panel get bogged down in a fruitless debate of personal points of view unsubstantiated by scientific evidence. He or she will strike a fine balance between letting the panellists "talk out" issues that seem to require a great deal of debate, and moving things along when further discussion is unlikely to produce any useful results. Throughout this process, the moderator will seek ways to encourage everyone to participate. Panellists are occasionally somewhat reticent at the beginning, as might be the case for general practitioners who are members of a panel composed primarily of specialists. Once the panellists become familiar with the process, however, there is usually no lack of discussion.

One way to start out the discussion might be to give panellists an overview of the results in a particular chapter or section. The moderator might say, for example, "You'll notice that for the indications in section x, you all pretty much agree that the procedure is appropriate for these patients, but in section y the ratings are less clear. What do you think is happening here?" Or, if the ratings for a particular indication are spread out over the whole scale (or concentrated at each end of the scale), panellists might be told, "If you'll look at indication number 12, you'll see that some people think the procedure is very appropriate, others think it is very inappropriate and still others are somewhere in the middle. There seems to be a lot of disagreement here. What is going on?" If no one volunteers anything at this point, the moderator might continue with "Do you think we have a problem of definition here? Are people perhaps thinking of different patients?" Or "Would any of the high (or low) raters like to explain why they rated that way?"

If the moderator notes that one person is consistently an outlier in rating a particular set of indications, an attempt may be made to include that person in the discussion to find out what was behind his thinking. This should be done by asking the panellist a non-threatening question, without indicating that this person is the outlier: for example, "What are your thoughts here?" or "How do you think one should approach a patient with this particular problem?" It is not a good idea to put anyone on the spot by directly asking "Why did you rate this indication differently from everybody else?" Sometimes the panellist may discover that the rating was simply an error; other times, he or she may maintain the difference of opinion with other panel members.

On all panels, there are some people who will participate much more actively in the discussion than others. This is normal and to be expected. However, there are ways to encourage more passive panel members to participate by, for example, directing a question at the table in general and then making eye contact with the person(s) whom one is trying to include in the discussion. One might also try to talk to the less active panellists during the coffee breaks to find out how they view the process and what might be impeding their participation. Reining in more aggressive participants is more delicate. *Avoiding* eye contact with them, calling on other panellists, and restating the opinions of other panellists are some non-obvious tactics to use. Actual confrontation will almost always cause more harm than good.

During the discussion, panellists should be encouraged to refer to the literature review with regard to issues that may be resolved by citing pertinent data. The moderator can set the tone for this by citing evidence from specific studies when it seems relevant to the discussion. In some cases, however, it may become evident that no amount of discussion will resolve the issue because there is no supporting scientific evidence. In such cases, the moderator should suggest that the panellists move on to another subject. It is important to keep good control of the time, realising that the first chapter or section of ratings invariably takes longer than those that follow. It may be necessary to remind the panel that they need to set a limit on the amount of discussion in order to be able to complete their work by the end of the specified period.

Sometimes panel discussions get bogged down in issues relating to how things are done in a particular practice or hospital. A panellist might say, "I understand that most physicians would recommend CABG for that patient, but in my hospital I would recommend the patient receive PTCA because the cardiovascular surgeons are very poor and we get excellent results using stents." Comments like this will prompt the moderator to remind the panellists that they are being asked to rate for an average patient presenting to an average physician who would recommend or perform the procedure in an average hospital. This is not to say that what they do in their particular settings is wrong, only that their appropriateness recommendations should not be based on unusual circumstances that are unlikely to apply to other clinical situations.

It may also be necessary to remind panellists at times that cost issues are not to be considered in their discussion or ratings. This can be difficult in some cases, for example, if they are rating the appropriateness of a procedure used for screening in the general population. It might help to remind the panellists that they are being asked to rate the *appropriateness* of the procedure, which does not necessarily mean that it *must* be done for all patients who fit the particular clinical scenario. That is, appropriateness and necessity are not the same thing: a procedure is appropriate when the benefits outweigh the risks; it is necessary when we would say it is wrong not to do it. For some procedures, such as CABG, it may well be that almost all appropriate indications are also necessary. For others, such as a diagnostic tool like gastrointestinal endoscopy, it may be that most of the appropriate indications are not necessary.

Cost is, of course, an important issue from a policy perspective or when a decision must be made as to what services a health service or system should pay for. However, once physicians agree that a procedure, test or treatment is *not inappropriate*, then further consideration can be given as to whether it should be covered. Other groups may need to participate in this decision, including consumers and policy-makers. Fortunately, the appropriateness ratings developed by expert physician panels have been found to agree rather well with cost-effectiveness models (Bernstein et al., 1997; Kuntz et al., 1999).

CHAPTER 8. CLASSIFYING APPROPRIATENESS

Introduction

In the RAND/UCLA appropriateness method a procedure is classified as
"appropriate," "uncertain" or "inappropriate" for a particular patient scenario
("indication") in accordance with 1) the *median* panel rating and 2) some measure
of the *dispersion* of panel ratings, which is taken as an indicator of the level of
agreement with which the ratings were made. Indications with median ratings in
the top third of the appropriateness scale are classified as appropriate, those with
median ratings in the bottom third are classified as inappropriate, and those with
intermediate median ratings are uncertain. In addition, indications for which the
dispersion of ratings is such as to indicate that the panellists disagree about
whether or not to recommend the procedure are also classified as uncertain. The
definitions used are discussed below.

Operational Definitions of Levels of Appropriateness

Indications are classified into three levels of appropriateness, using the
following definitions:

- *Appropriate*: panel median of 7-9, without disagreement
- *Uncertain*: panel median of 4-6 OR any median with disagreement
- *Inappropriate*: panel median of 1-3, without disagreement

These definitions can be applied to any rating done by an odd number of
raters. If there are an even number of panellists, it is possible to have decimal
medians, therefore a decision must be made about how to treat median ratings
that fall exactly between the 3-point boundaries, that is, medians of 3.5 and 6.5.
The most common approach (which is biased towards making indications
appropriate and thus favours physician autonomy) includes these medians in the
higher appropriateness category, so that a median of 6.5 would be appropriate, and
one of 3.5 would be uncertain. Alternatively, a "round to the middle" strategy
would assign both cases to the uncertain category.

Operational Definitions of Levels of Disagreement

The key issue, then, is what constitutes *disagreement*. Various approaches
have been used in an attempt to establish definitions that most people would

accept as reasonable. Definitions of *agreement* have also been developed (Park et al., 1986), but in practice these are rarely used, since the appropriateness classification depends only on the median and the presence or absence of disagreement. We include definitions of agreement in this manual for completeness and in case a user of the RAM might wish to employ the concept. In the early years of the RAM, various alternative definitions were developed , the so-called "strict" and "relaxed" definitions (Table 3).

Table 3. Strict versus Relaxed Definitions of *Agreement* and *Disagreement* for 9-Member Panels

Definition	Meaning
Agreement	
• A9S*	All nine ratings fall within a single 3-point region (1-3; 4-6; 7-9).
• A9R†	All nine ratings fall within any 3-point range.
• A7S	After discarding one extreme high and one extreme low rating, the remaining seven ratings all fall within a single 3-point region (1-3; 4-6; 7-9).
• A7R	After discarding one extreme high and one extreme low rating, the remaining seven ratings all fall within any 3-point range.
Disagreement	
• D9S	Considering all nine ratings, at least one is a 1, and at least one is a 9.
• D9R	Considering all nine ratings, at least one falls in the lowest 3-point region (1-3), and at least one falls in the highest (7-9).
• D7S	After discarding one extreme high and one extreme low rating, at least one of the remaining seven ratings is a 1, and at least one is a 9. ‡
• D7R	After discarding one extreme high and one extreme low rating, at least one of the remaining seven ratings falls in the lowest 3-point region (1-3), and at least one falls in the highest (7-9). ‡

* S = Strict
† R = Relaxed
‡ Note that this is the same as at least two ratings at one extreme and at least two ratings at the other.
Source: Brook et al., 1986

Applying these and other definitions to different data sets, the RAND researchers settled on what has been termed the "classic" definition for a 9-member panel, as it is the one that has most commonly been applied:

- **Agreement:** No more than 2 panellists rate the indication outside the 3-point region (1-3; 4-6; 7-9) containing the median.
- **Disagreement:** At least three panellists rate the indication in the 1-3 region, and at least three panellists rate it in the 7-9 region.

In an attempt to anticipate the problem of how to deal with panels composed of more or fewer than nine members, RAND translated the preceding definitions into a "somewhat statistical" form, framed as tests of hypotheses about the distribution of ratings in a hypothetical population of repeated ratings by similarly selected panellists (Leape et al., 1991):

- **Agreement**: "We test the hypothesis that 80 percent of the hypothetical population of repeated ratings are within the same region (1-3, 4-6, 7-9) as the observed median. If we are unable to reject that hypothesis on a binomial test at the 0.33 level, we say that the indication is rated 'with agreement'."
- **Disagreement**. "We test the hypothesis that 90 percent of the hypothetical population of repeated ratings are within one of two extra wide regions (1-6 or 4-9). If we have to reject that hypothesis on a binomial test at the 0.10 level, we conclude that the indication is rated 'with disagreement'."

This solution, however, also presented difficulties. If disagreement is to be defined in terms of the number of ratings at each extreme of the scale, there are only a limited number of possibilities since panellists can only be thought of in terms of whole numbers: 2, 3, 4 or 5, depending on the panel size. The multinational European panels carried out as part of the BIOMED Concerted Action on Appropriateness, which each invited 15 panel members to participate, planned for this contingency by agreeing beforehand to adopt the definitions shown in Table 4.

Table 4. Definitions of *Agreement* and *Disagreement* for Different Panel Sizes

Panel Size	*Disagreement* Number of panellists rating in each extreme (1-3 and 7-9)	*Agreement* Number of panellists rating outside the 3-point region containing the median (1-3; 4-6; 7-9)
8-9-10	≥ 3	≤ 2
11-12-13	≥ 4	≤ 3
14-15-16	≥ 5	≤ 4

The definitions of *agreement* shown in the preceding table follow logically from the definitions of *disagreement*: the minimum number of panellists permitted to rate outside the region containing the median must be *one less* than the number of panellists rating in the extremes for disagreement; otherwise the two definitions would not be mutually exclusive. These definitions, however, are still not entirely satisfactory. They work well for panels that are multiples of three, because the definition of *disagreement* is the same: at least one-third of the panellists rate in each extreme. Within each group, however, the definition of *disagreement* will be biased, producing less disagreement for the smallest panels and more disagreement for the largest.

A New Approach to Measuring Disagreement

Given the problems discussed in the preceding section, one of the objectives of the BIOMED Concerted Action on Appropriateness was to develop and test new definitions of *disagreement* that could easily be applied to any panel size. Investigators at the *Unidad de Investigación en Servicios de Salud* (UISS) of the Carlos III Health Institute in Madrid have been working on such a measure, which it was agreed should meet the following criteria:

- The measure should be continuous.
- It should be possible to apply it to any size panel.
- The results of applying the measure should be consistent with those produced by applying the classic definition to panels that are multiples of 3.
- It should be possible to move the cut-off point to test stricter and more relaxed definitions of agreement and disagreement.

The only continuous measure that has been used to date has been the mean absolute deviation from the median (MAD-M). Some appropriateness panels include this statistic on their panellist forms, but it is rarely used except, perhaps, by some moderators as a guide to what indications to focus on during the panel discussion. The new measure developed is based on the Interpercentile Range (IPR), which is a commonly-used statistical measure of dispersion of a distribution and seemed a reasonable candidate for exploration.

Development of the "IPRAS"

Experiments were made comparing the indications labelled as disagreement by the classic definition to those so labelled with the new measure. This was done using data from panels that were multiples of 3 (that is, 9, 12 or 15 panellists). The best results (those closest to the classic method) were found with an IPR of 0.3 - 0.7 (calculated using Microsoft Excel).

In-depth examination of the cases of disagreement identified by the IPR led to an interesting discovery: when the ratings were symmetric with respect to the middle (5 on the 1-9 scale), the IPR required to label an indication as disagreement was smaller than when the ratings were asymmetric with respect to the middle (values far from 5 on the 1-9 scale). Based on this finding another measure was developed, which has been named IPRAS (Interpercentile Range Adjusted for Symmetry). The rationale behind it is that when ratings are symmetric, the IPR required to label an indication as disagreement is smaller than when they are asymmetric.

Asymmetry was defined as "the distance between the central point of the IPR and the central point of the 1-9 scale, i.e. 5." Since the more asymmetric the ratings are, the larger is the IPR required to say that there is disagreement, the following mathematical function was developed:

$$IPRAS = IPRr + (AI * CFA), \text{ where}$$

IPRAS is the Interpercentile Range Adjusted for Symmetry required for disagreement;

IPRr is the Interpercentile Range required for disagreement when perfect symmetry exists;

AI is the Asymmetry Index; and

CFA is the Correction Factor for Asymmetry.

Thus, each indication requires a different IPRAS to be classified as disagreement, depending on its internal symmetry. Consequently, indication i is rated with disagreement if

$$IPR_i > IPRAS_i.$$

The values that best reproduce the "classic" definitions in the data sets applied are:

IPRr = 2.35

CFA = 1.5

Thus, the final formula is:

$$IPRAS = 2.35 + (AI * 1.5)$$

In summary, if the IPR of a particular indication is larger than the IPRAS of that particular indication, the indication is rated with disagreement. Applying this definition to different data sets, we can obtain false positives (FP)—indications labelled disagreement by the IPRAS but not by the classic definition—and false negatives (FN)—indications labelled disagreement by the classic definition but not by the IPRAS. (Note that in the present context, *positive = disagreement*).

The IPRAS yielded a sensitivity of 1 in almost all data sets tested, with a good specificity. Initially the IPRAS was tested in a total of 5,566 indications from 6 data sets. Twenty-one FN and 75 FP were obtained. Exploring each of these discordant indications, it was found that one advantage of the IPRAS in comparison to the classic definition is that it smoothes the rigid frontier between 3-4 and 6-7, and is a better measure of the degree of dispersion among ratings. This advantage would seem to solve one of the limitations of the classic definition that has been observed previously: that is, there are some indications for which panellist ratings are widely scattered across almost all categories, and yet they do not meet the classic definition of disagreement ("FP" cases). The opposite situation also occurs, but rarely: cases in which the classic definition says that there is disagreement and the IPRAS does not, ("FN" cases). These tend to be ratings that are highly asymmetric, but with the bulk of the ratings falling at one or another extreme of the scale, so that one might question if this really constitutes "disagreement".

Two examples from a panel of 12 panellists illustrate the foregoing:

Example 1:

Frequencies 3 1 2   4   2

Rating scale 1 2 3 4 5 6 7 8 9

There are 6 ratings in the 1-3 range and 2 ratings in the 7-9 range. As a result, according to the classic method there is no disagreement. The IPRAS method works as follows:

The Lp (Lower limit IPR) is 2.3; the Up (Upper limit IPR) is 6.0; thus, the IPR is 3.7.

The IPRCP (Central point of IPR) is 4.15 ((2.3+6.0)/2).

The Asymmetry Index is 0.85 (5-4.15).

Thus, the IPRAS is 2.35 + (1.5 * Asymmetry Index)= 3.63.

Since IPR (3.7) > IPRAS (3.63), there **is disagreement**.

In the preceding example, we can see that six panellists rated in the 1-3 range and six panellists in the 6-8 range. The IPRAS is sensitive to this kind of dispersion (disagreement), whereas the classic method is not.

Example 2:

Frequencies 2 2 4   3 1

Rating scale 1 2 3 4 5 6 7 8 9

In example 2, there are 8 ratings in the 1-3 range and 4 ratings in the 7-9 range. As a result, according to the classic method there is disagreement. With IPRAS calculations:

The Lp (Lower limit IPR) is 2.3; the Up (Upper limit IPR) is 5.8; thus, the IPR is 3.5.

The IPRCP (Central point of IPR) is 4.05 ((2.3+5.8)/2)

The Asymmetry Index is 0.95 (5-4.05)

Thus, the IPRAS is 2.35 + (1.5 * Asymmetry Index)= 3.78.

Since IPR (3.5) < IPRAS (3.78), there is **no disagreement**.

In this example, we can see that eight panellists rated in the 1-3 range and four panellists in the 7-8 range. Thus, two thirds of the panellists are concentrated at the lower end of the scale (inappropriate). The IPRAS is sensitive to this kind of weight in the extremes (disagreement), whereas the classic method looks only at whether or not one third of the ratings are in each 3-point extreme of the scale.

The IPRAS has now been tested in a variety of data sets: 7 real panels and 4 simulated panels, totalling more than 16,400 theoretical indications and more than 6,500 real cases. Only a very small number of cases of discrepancies have been found with comparison to the classic definition. Close examination of such cases by a number of investigators involved in different appropriateness projects has shown that the IPRAS classification seems to make more logical sense than the classic definition. Persons wishing more information on this subject are encouraged to contact the research group at the Carlos III Health Institute where the method was developed (see Annex I).

CHAPTER 9. SOFTWARE TOOLS FOR DATA PROCESSING AND ANALYSIS

Introduction

A key issue confronting all researchers planning an appropriateness project is how to process the large volume of data resulting from the rating process. The main tasks involved are: 1) creating the indications list for the first round ratings; 2) producing the customised panellist documents for the second (and possibly third) round ratings, together with the two moderator documents; and 3) producing the statistical analyses in a variety of formats. If the appropriateness criteria are to be applied to a patient population to measure overuse (or underuse), additional programs must be designed to collect data from clinical records, classify each patient in accordance with the list of indications, and identify the corresponding appropriateness rating for that indication.

While these general objectives are shared by all appropriateness projects, the approaches adopted in specific projects vary widely depending on the available software and expertise of the information specialists involved. One lesson learned from the BIOMED Concerted Action project is that no "generic" software is needed to deal with all possible lists of indications. There have been many solutions proposed to the problem of generating the documents needed, and experience has shown that they all work reasonably well. In particular, software developed at RAND in Santa Monica, as well as versions by the Concerted Action partners Carlos III Health Institute (Madrid), Erasmus University (Rotterdam), the Institute of Social and Preventive Medicine (Lausanne) and Mario Negri Institute (Milan) all may be recommended for use. Information on how to contact the various groups that have produced software packages can be found in Annex I.

Anyone planning to carry out an appropriateness panel should be aware, however, that specific resources must be designated to data processing needs. The degree of specialisation involved may be quite variable—from persons with advanced knowledge of a commonly used program such as Excel, to information specialists capable of programming in such sophisticated languages as JAVA. Since a number of different capabilities are required (printing out forms, data base and statistical analysis), some projects have used a different program to perform each task, for example, word processing software to produce the rating forms and a statistical package for data analysis. The following sections give a brief summary of some of the software approaches that have been adopted in different appropriateness projects.

RAND, Santa Monica, California

The earliest RAND projects used SAS and STATA, two packages that include capabilities making it possible to perform all the tasks enumerated in the preceding sections. These programs have several characteristics that make them both powerful and versatile:

- They include many of the most advanced statistical procedures as well as myriad functions for handling numeric and text data.
- Programs can be written using simple syntax.
- They have capabilities for editing and printing results in a user-designed format.
- SAS has a query language (SQL) which makes it possible to "cross" the data produced by the panellists with those collected from the clinical records.

Other statistical packages, such as SPSS, share many of these same capabilities and are likely to serve equally well; however, there has been little experience in using them for appropriateness projects.

Erasmus University, Rotterdam

The investigators at Erasmus University relied on a programming language known as Delphi ("Visual Pascal") to produce the forms needed for their appropriateness panels. One program is used to generate the blank ratings booklets for use in the first round. The core of the program is simply a nested loop, with the loop variables representing the values of the clinical factors (for example, the variable "age" might have two values: <70 years and $\geq$70 years). Another program calculates the median ratings, as well as the agreement and appropriateness classifications, and is used to generate the customised ratings booklets for the second round; this program highlights the panellist's individual score in red.

Delphi is a very flexible tool, but a substantial amount of programming was involved. Moreover, not everything can be done in Delphi. It was necessary to import the "rough" forms into a word processor and clean them up. The statistical analysis for the Dutch panels was performed using SPSS for Windows.

Carlos III Health Institute, Madrid

The Madrid project has shown how relatively simple software tools can be used to produce results quite similar to those of more sophisticated programs. A spreadsheet is basically a program to store data in a matrix structure, where each observation is identified by its corresponding row and column. In general, working with a spreadsheet gives the user the agreeable feeling that both the data and the results are readily accessible. The structure of the list of indications can be modified quite easily, by adding or eliminating rows or columns. Spreadsheets incorporate an extensive catalogue of arithmetic and statistical functions, which facilitate the statistical analysis of panellist ratings. They also have some data base functions, but these are more limited than in a strictly data base program such as Access or dBase. Learning to use these types of programs is relatively quick and simple, however, designing the overall program requires advanced knowledge of spreadsheet functions.

In the Madrid approach, the program for data entry and analysis consists of multiple "sheets" within an Excel "book." For example, the first two sheets are used for dual entry of the panellist ratings (in columns), while the third sheet highlights any discrepancies in data entry. A fourth sheet contains the median for each indication, the frequencies for each three point interval (1-3; 4-6; 7-9), and the agreement and appropriateness classification. Additional sheets are used to generate the panellist and moderator documents and tables of the results. It is also possible to carry out different types of analysis, for example, to compare the effect of different definitions of "disagreement" on the appropriateness classifications.

Institute of Social and Preventive Medicine, University of Lausanne

In planning the European panel on gastrointestinal endoscopy, the Lausanne investigators decided to use JAVA for their software needs. This decision was influenced by two important constraints imposed by the research group:

- The application had to allow for smooth transition of data from the panel to an experimental web site used to present data.

- It had to allow near real-time analysis of the second round (appropriateness) data and preparation of forms for the third round (necessity) ratings. This was required so that both appropriateness and necessity could be rated at the same panel meeting.

JAVA is the most advanced tool for software development. It is an object-oriented program, that is, applications called "applets" are developed to carry out each task, which is independent of other tasks. An applet, once designed, can be used in any program. Moreover, all software needed to run the application is in the public domain and the application itself is compact, with a size of only 100 KB. JAVA owes much of its prestige to the Internet, where it is rapidly becoming a standard. This means that applications written in this language may be quite easy to disseminate through the network. This undoubtedly constitutes an additional advantage, since panel results could be disseminated very rapidly to interested parties. A disadvantage of the application, at least in its present form, is that it is not user-friendly for the novice, although it can easily be mastered in an hour's time for someone with moderate computer literacy.

The Swiss JAVA-based program generates both HTML and ASCII based pages of the panel ratings forms. Input files are text files of the columns and rows of the indications matrices and a flat data file of panel ratings. The output files are the usual RAND panel matrix: blank forms for the first round ratings, moderator forms and customised panellist forms with the results of the first round ratings, and the final appropriateness criteria based on the results of the second round ratings. In addition, the program permits immediate generation of the forms required for the third round (necessity) ratings.

The files with the final appropriateness and necessity criteria can also be used, with minor adjustments, for the experimental web site that the Lausanne group has developed to allow easy access to panel results (see Chapter 12). This website is publicly available at www.epage.ch. Further advantages of the JAVA approach are that all software needed to run the application is in the public domain and the application itself is compact, with a size of only 100 KB.

Data entry was performed with a separate program.

CHAPTER 10. APPLYING APPROPRIATENESS CRITERIA RETROSPECTIVELY TO MEASURE OVERUSE

Introduction

Appropriateness criteria, originally developed to measure retrospectively the overuse of a procedure, can be used in a number of ways, including retrospective examination of underuse, prospective examination of overuse and underuse, construction of guidelines or decision aids to help physicians decide whether to perform a procedure for a particular patient, or determining the most needed clinical studies with respect to a procedure. In this chapter, we review the original use, which was the retrospective employment of medical chart audits to determine the proportion of patients in a study population who received a procedure considered to be "appropriate," "uncertain," or "inappropriate." This chapter gives a broad overview of some of the factors that should be considered when planning a study designed to use appropriateness ratings in this way.

Before beginning a research project of this type, the investigators will need to make some basic decisions about the population to which the criteria will be applied, the resources that will be required, and the method of data collection. Some of the issues involved in each decision are discussed below:

- *The study population.* Appropriateness criteria should be applied to the population and the time period for which they were designed.   Thus, criteria developed by a Spanish panel of experts in coronary revascularization should be applied to Spanish patients who were revascularized in approximately the same time period as when the criteria were developed. The length of time the criteria remain current will depend largely on what new studies have been released or new technological innovations have been introduced since they were developed.

- *Economic and logistical limitations.* The available time, budget, and human resources are critical factors affecting the field work as they will determine the size and design of the study.   Whereas a national level audit could be made with as few as 500 cases, the design of a sampling frame for such an audit and obtaining the cooperation of the necessary centers might be a logistical nightmare. Many more cases will be needed if the study is intended to detect possible differences among individual centers or geographic regions. A local level examination can be done much more quickly and economically—however, the results may not be generalizable.

- *Data availability.* The information needed to classify patients in accordance with the list of indications must be accessible to the researcher. The usual sources of data in studies of medical procedures are patient charts or records. It is necessary to assure, first, that authorisation can be obtained to access the charts, second, that they can be easily located, and third, that they contain sufficient information to classify each patient. Depending on the type of institutional review procedures established to govern research involving human subjects, it may be necessary to obtain formal approval from a review board or committee to collect this type of data. At times it may be necessary to obtain information directly from the patient if it is not available in the medical record. This can pose a particular challenge if one needs to assess the impact of the patient's condition on functional status or quality of life (Rowe et al., 1999; Broder et al., 2000).

To measure overuse, all that is basically needed are the appropriateness criteria and the population, usually relatively circumscribed, of those patients who have received the procedure. Applying the criteria to those cases will give us an idea of how many are inappropriate (see Figure 17).

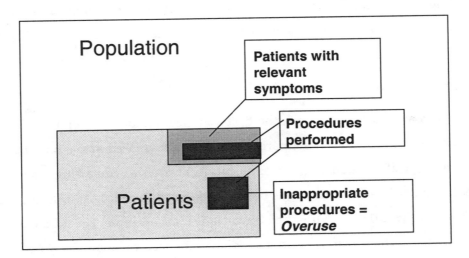

Figure 17. Overuse of Procedures. *Cases of overuse of a procedure (i.e., those that are inappropriate) are to be found among the population of patients who have received the procedure.*

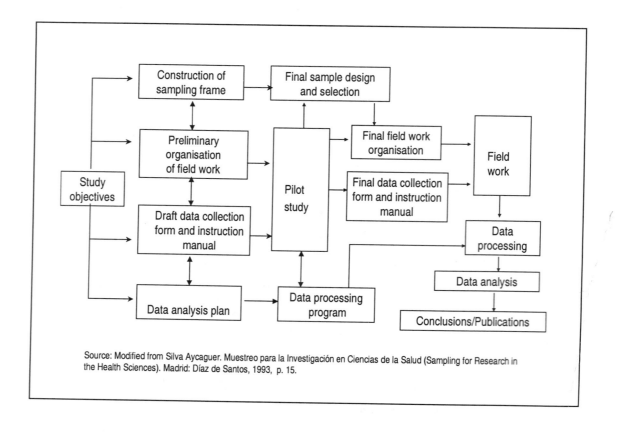

Figure 18. Design of a Retrospective Study to Measure Appropriateness

Figure 18 shows an outline of the steps involved in carrying out a typical retrospective appropriateness survey. Each of these steps is discussed briefly in the following sections.

Study Objectives

As in any research project, the first and most important step is to define the objectives of the study. Will appropriateness be measured at the national level, or within a specific region or group of hospitals, or even within a single hospital or health centre? Will comparisons be made among different hospitals or geographic regions, or by different patient characteristics (for example, age, sex, clinical conditions)? The specific objectives of the study need to be precisely defined as they will determine the size of the study and the resources required to carry it out.

Construction of the Sampling Frame

Target population. The size of the target population can vary greatly, as one may be interested in measuring appropriateness in a single hospital or a group of hospitals, or the project may have the more ambitious goal of measuring appropriateness throughout an entire region or country.

Time period of the study. Appropriateness criteria are developed in accordance with the technological reality at a particular point in time, and should be applied accordingly. It would not make sense to apply appropriateness criteria for PTCA that were developed when intra-coronary artery stents were in widespread use to a population of patients who were revascularized before this technology was available. Likewise, there is no point in trying to measure appropriateness using criteria that have become obsolete because of new scientific evidence or the introduction of superior treatment modalities. The rapid advances in medical knowledge and technology constitute one of the major challenges to the RAM, as appropriateness criteria can quickly become outdated. Some possible solutions to this problem are discussed in Chapter 13.

Sample size. It is usually not possible to measure appropriateness in the entire target population. Normally, a representative sample of the population is selected and appropriateness rates in the population are estimated based on the sample results. Different formulas to calculate sample sizes can be found in many textbooks, but they all require knowledge of the following parameters:

- The *total number of procedures* carried out during the specified time period in the geographic area of study. This is usually the most difficult information to obtain, especially when the target population is large and geographically disperse. Often there is no reliable database to determine the number of procedures carried out, and it may be necessary to consult several sources or to assume the number as infinite.

- An estimate of the *expected proportion of inappropriate use.* Information from previous studies or the results of the pilot test may be used for this estimate. Alternatively, one can assume that it is 50%, the least advantageous case which will result in a larger sample size than any other estimate.

- The *maximum acceptable error* in the estimate of the proportion of inappropriate use. This figure indicates the required precision of the final results. The smaller the error, the more precise the final results, but the larger the sample size.

- The *confidence level* for the measurement. As in the case of maximum error, the higher the confidence level, the larger the sample size. Traditionally, most studies use a 95% confidence level.

Type of sample. The ideal sample is a random sample in which all of the elements (units of analysis) have some probability of forming part of the sample and this probability is known for each element. In a simple random sample, each element has the same probability of being included. This type of sampling facilitates calculations of sampling error when making inferences about the entire population. Simple random sampling may be feasible when the target population is geographically concentrated in a relatively small number of areas. When the target population is dispersed, however, it is often divided into clusters to facilitate sampling logistics. Clusters may consist of a single set of units of analysis (single-stage sampling) or two or more such sets (two-stage or multi-stage sampling). In studies of medical procedures in large geographical areas, a first-stage cluster could be a hospital or health region, while a second-stage cluster could be a particular department within the hospital or a health centre. Clusters can be selected by simple random sampling, with each cluster having the same probability of being included in the sample, or the probability of selection can be made proportional to the size of the cluster if they are very unequal in size. The final units of analysis—in the case of the RAM, patient charts—are selected from the last-stage clusters.

Random selection of the units of analysis or even of the clusters does not guarantee that the sample will be representative of the entire population. If the analysis is to be made with reference to specific factors that are thought to affect appropriateness rates, such as the volume of procedures performed, then it may be desirable to stratify the sample accordingly (for example, hospitals performing fewer than 100 procedures per year, those performing 100-300 and those performing more than 300). Care should be taken not to overstratify, however, or there may not be enough units of analysis in each stratum to permit subsequent analysis.

The preceding comments do not pretend to be a substantive guide to sample design, but only to alert the investigator to the importance of answering certain questions about the target population at the beginning of the study: How many units of analysis are there? How are they distributed geographically? How will the possible factors related with appropriateness be identified? Only when these questions have been resolved can the statistician design the sample that best fits the needs and limitations of the project.

Preliminary Organisation of Field Work

The cost and complexity of the field work is directly proportional to the size of the sample. The major questions that need to be resolved in planning the field work are discussed below.

Accessing the source of information. It is not always easy to obtain the collaboration of persons outside the project when making a retrospective chart audit. However, if the sample is truly to be representative of the larger population it is important that all or almost all centres agree to participate. If there is an appreciable refusal or "non-response" rate, the possible bias introduced could call into question the validity of the study results.

Data collection. Who will collect the data? How many persons will be necessary? Will they be paid and, if so, how much? The answers to these questions will depend on the size of the study and the financial and human resources available for the project. In whatever case, it is essential to hold a training session for the persons responsible for data collection (sometimes referred to as "abstractors" in appropriateness studies). Trained clinical nurse abstractors are probably the best choice for a study in which the data source is clinical charts, but other health professionals such as medical residents could also be used. At the training session the study investigators should explain the clinical issue being studied and how the data required to assess appropriateness is to be collected. It is important to give the abstractors an opportunity to review sample charts and to provide them with a detailed "how-to" manual as well as definitions of the study terms. The number of abstractors required depends directly on how long it takes to fill out each form, and inversely on the amount of time they can dedicate to this task and the duration of the data collection period. If resources permit, a fixed amount should be paid for each completed form; incomplete forms or those meeting exclusion criteria are not compensated. The most critical aspect is the quality and completeness of the information that exists in the medical records. This may vary by the topic under investigation. Thus, while an early study conducted in the US indicated that medical records were a valid source of information for classifying the appropriateness of coronary angiography (Kosecoff et al., 1987), a recent study in Switzerland concluded that the information retrievable from patient medical records was insufficient to classify patients for the appropriateness of lumbar disc surgery (Jeannot et al., 1999). The Spanish experience was mixed: in a national sample of patients undergoing coronary revascularization it was possible to classify the great majority of patients, although it was sometimes necessary to make certain assumptions in the face of missing data, always in the direction of favouring appropriateness (MD Aguilar, unpublished data). The quality of medical records may well vary among different countries.

Identifying the units of analysis. To construct a random sample (n), it is necessary to have a list of all the units of analysis in the total population (N). The units of analysis to be included in the sample are then chosen by selecting n random numbers from N, using a statistical package or table of random numbers. When cluster sampling is involved (health services or centres), the random selection is made for each cluster.

Control of duplicates. The unit of analysis may be the patient or the procedure. Since it is possible that the same patient may undergo the procedure more than once, a decision needs to be made on how to handle such cases.

Sampling with replacement. Some charts selected in the sample cannot be included in the study, either because they meet one of the exclusion criteria (for example, the procedure was not done on the patient) or they cannot be located. In such cases, it may be possible to select a replacement chart if the principle of random selection can be maintained without introducing bias. This can be done by providing the abstractors with a "replacement list" of random numbers. The abstractors should receive clear instructions in the training session and in the manual about when and how to select a replacement chart. The reason for replacement should be clearly specified in each case. The investigators should exercise caution, however, if a large number of charts cannot be located: if the probability of an inappropriate procedure is higher for patients whose charts are missing, the rate of inappropriate use will be underestimated in the study population.

Field work co-ordination. The field work should be organised and directed by someone with previous experience in this type of study. It is important to have a good infrastructure for communications, i.e., telephone, fax and email capabilities. The time required for this phase of the project will depend on the sample size, the number of participating centres and the number of abstractors involved. As an example, a Spanish national-level study of the appropriateness of coronary revascularization required one full-time and another half-time person working for 6 months to co-ordinate a review of 4000 patient charts in 30 centres with 42 chart abstractors.

Mailing the forms. The abstractors should be given a timetable for returning the forms. For example, they may be asked to return them in sets of 20 or 50, or to send all the forms completed each week. They should receive precise instructions on how to mail the forms, preferably by courier service or certified mail, in case lost packages need to be traced.

Contacts with abstractors. The data abstractors, and their supervisors, should be able to contact the data co-ordinator at specified times to resolve possible problems. All such contacts should be documented, showing when they occurred, the reason for the contact, and the action to be taken. The field work co-ordinator should contact each abstractor after receiving the first set of data collection forms or whenever a problem is detected, both to provide information about the quality of the data collection and to motivate the abstractor to continue.

Quality control. Certain mechanisms can be built into the database to control the quality of the information contained in the data collection forms. Thus, it is important to enter the data as the forms are received so that those not meeting the quality tests can be returned to the abstractor for correction. The forms should be kept in a place easily accessible to the field work co-ordinator, and classified in a way that permits easy localisation of any form that needs to be rechecked.

Ideally, some charts (e.g., 5% of the study sample) should be abstracted twice by two different people to check inter-abstractor reliability. If duplicate data abstraction cannot be done in the field, it is important to have abstractors practice abstracting a sufficient number of charts to assure a reasonable level of inter-abstractor reliability (see "Pilot Study" in this chapter).

Overreading. For some appropriateness studies, abstractors may not have sufficient knowledge or skills to correctly classify some patient variables. In this case, they may be asked to copy information from the medical record verbatim and/or to photocopy portions of the medical record or test results for coding by a physician at study headquarters.

Draft Data Collection Form and Instruction Manual

The data collection form is the instrument used to extract the information needed for the study from the medical charts. The basic requirements of any such form are that it be valid, that is, it should correctly measure what it intends to measure, and reliable, that is, it should consistently produce the same results when used with the same data source.

Data collection forms may contain three different types of questions:

- *Closed* questions, in which the choice of responses is listed on the form. Care should be taken to assure that the response categories chosen include all possible replies, including "information not available" or "unknown".
- *Open* questions, in which the abstractors write in their own reply.
- *Quantitative* questions, in which the answer is a number, for example an age or birth-date. Some quantitative questions use a scale for the respondent to reply.

In data processing, closed and quantitative questions are easier to interpret than open ones.

Some general recommendations in developing a data collection instrument are as follows:

- All the questions should relate to the objectives of the research project.
- Questions should be clearly formulated, using simple language and avoiding ambiguities.
- It should be easy to answer the questions using the information routinely found in the data sources.
- A correctly completed form should allow classification of the patient into one (and only one) indication in the list of indications.

An instruction manual should accompany the data collection form so the abstractors can refer to it during the data collection process. The manual should include general instructions on how to fill out the form and specific instructions on each question that will anticipate and resolve possible problems or confusion. Where appropriate, precise definitions of terms used in the form should also be included. It is essential to test the form, the instruction manual, and the classification program in a pilot study.

Some studies have examined patient cases prospectively, for example, by recording the requested information at the time the medical procedure is performed. This requires the collaboration of the person in charge of the procedure (usually a physician) and is more likely to assure that all the information necessary to classify the patient in the indications list is recorded. The key question is to have a questionnaire that is comprehensive, while still being of manageable length.

Data Analysis Plan

In planning the data analysis, it is important to consider how the data are to be used to meet the study objectives and what variables will need to be included in the tables of the final report. This subject should be considered before producing the form, so that all the necessary variables will be included.

Data Processing Program

Frequently, the questions on the form do not permit direct classification of the patient in the list of indications, therefore it is necessary to write a program to transform the data into the variables necessary for classification. For example, a form designed to measure the appropriateness of coronary revascularization would require many different questions to classify a patient's stress test results as "positive" "negative," etc., in accordance with the definitions used by the expert panel in making their judgements. Decisions may need to be made about which test results take priority, in the event that a patient has received several tests.

In a Spanish study of the appropriateness of coronary revascularization, the data collection form included more than 200 data elements. The data transformation program reduced these to the 12 variables needed to classify each patient according to the list of indications. A simplified example of this process is shown in Figure 19.

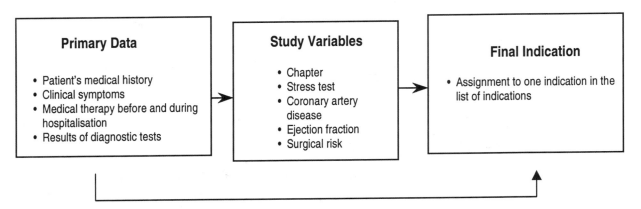

Figure 19 Transformation of Variables

Pilot Study

Before beginning the actual field work, a pilot study should be performed under circumstances similar to those in which the final field work will be carried out: the abstractors should have the same qualifications and the same data sources should be used.   This step is essential for the detection of potential problems and modification of the study protocol when it is still relatively easy to do so. The main objectives of the pilot study are:

- *To test the training session for the data abstractors*. The questions raised during the pilot training session may lead to revision of the data collection form or instruction manual. The training session may also give the investigator an idea of how enthusiastic the participants are, and whether new strategies to motivate them need to be designed.

- *To test the field-work control mechanisms*. This includes the plan for how forms will be registered when they are sent to the field work co-ordinator, control of data entry, documentation of "missing" items, and contacts with abstractors to obtain missing information whenever possible.

- *To validate the data collection form and instruction manual*. The pilot study will show whether the questions can be answered with the information typically available in patient charts. For example, the pilot study may show that charts in private hospitals do not include complete information about the medications the patient is taking, therefore it may not be possible to know whether these patients were on "optimal" or "sub-optimal" medical therapy before the procedure. A decision needs to be made about how these patients will be treated. Will they be excluded from the study? Will it be assumed that they were on optimal medical therapy, to avoid biasing against appropriateness? Any such assumptions need to be clearly stated in the report of the study as they will affect the reader's interpretation of the results.

- *To measure the reliability of the data collection instrument*, as well *as intra- and inter-observer reliability*. Intra-observer reliability can be measured by having the same person fill out the form using the same data source on two different occasions (at least one month apart). The abstractors should not be told ahead of time that they may be asked to do this. Inter-observer reliability is measured by having two different persons fill out the data collection form from the same patient charts, then measuring the inter-observer agreement. Both intra- and inter-observer reliability can be improved by training the abstractors and providing them with an easy-to-use and complete instruction manual. Inclusion of a test of inter-observer reliability in the pilot study can be very helpful in improving the reliability of the data collection form. Questions with a low level of inter-observer agreement may need to be reworded to eliminate subjectivity; alternatively it may be that the data source simply does not provide enough data to allow an objective response to the question. The comments and suggestions of the abstractors in the pilot study are also very helpful in improving the reliability of the data collection form since it is in the field where inconsistencies are most easily detected.

- *To assure that the patient can be assigned to a specific indication*. The pilot test is also used to confirm if enough data is available to classify the patient in accordance with the list of indications. The pilot may show that some questions are superfluous since they are not used to classify patients, therefore they may be eliminated. On the other hand, it may also be found that additional questions are needed to enable patient classification.

- *To validate the data transformation program* used to assign the patient to a specific indication.

- *To calculate the percentage of charts with enough information to classify the patient in the list of indications*. If this percentage is substantially different from the assumptions used in calculating the sample size, it may be necessary to recalculate the sample size to maintain the same precision and confidence level chosen for the estimate.

Final Sample Design and Selection

The final design of the sample will depend on having obtained answers to the questions raised in the previous steps: the definition of the population, its geographical distribution, if/how it is to be stratified, the type of sample, the percentage of charts lacking sufficient information to be classified in the list of indications, and the percentage of inappropriate procedures in the pilot study. Persons lacking knowledge of sampling techniques should consult an expert in this area.

Final Field Work Organisation

Much of the organisational work will have been accomplished by incorporating the modifications suggested by the pilot study. At this point, the mechanisms to carry out and control the final field work should be well established.

In preparing for contacts with the centres selected for the final sample, it is important to consider how they can be motivated to participate. It is understandable that some hospitals may be reluctant to be part of a study that is designed to show what proportion of procedures have been performed for inappropriate or uncertain reasons. Some points to be emphasised in contacts with the persons responsible for authorising the study in each centre may help to alleviate their concern about how the study results are to be used:

- Explain the study objectives clearly, emphasising that the validity of the results will depend on having complete participation in the study.
- Provide background information on how the appropriateness criteria were developed and how the study is being financed. Emphasise that the study is being done not as a way to reduce costs, but to improve individual patient care.
- Make sure the centres understand exactly what effort is being requested of them (number of abstractors, hours of time required, if they are to be paid).
- Offer each centre the possibility of receiving their own individual data, while assuring them that their data will remain confidential and will not be linked by name with the centre.

If the study is well designed and clearly explained to the centres, if they are assured of the confidentiality of their individual data, and if they will have access to their own data, they are much more likely to participate.

Final Data Collection Form and Instruction Manual

After analysing the pilot study and the suggestions of the data abstractors in the pilot training session, the corresponding modifications will be made to the data collection form and instruction manual.

Field Work

As in the pilot study, the first step is to train the data abstractors. The training session will be based on the experience acquired in the pilot test, incorporating the improvements suggested in the data collection form, instruction manual and training session itself. Data should be entered as the forms are received as this will facilitate detection of problems in time to resolve them. Abstractors should be informed immediately as to any errors of conception or interpretation detected so they can be corrected, and similar errors can be avoided in the remaining forms. Precise instructions should be provided as to when the forms are to be mailed: perhaps every 10 to 20 forms, depending on their length, complexity and the number assigned to each abstractor.

It may prove difficult to obtain all the completed forms within the period planned for data collection. Intensive follow-up will help assure that late responders meet their commitment to fill out the specified number of forms. It is better to extend the data collection period a few extra weeks than to risk losing those forms which are hardest to obtain since this could result in major bias to the study. The real end of the data collection period is when the last form has been entered in the database, all corrections have been made, and any problems with the abstractors have been resolved.

Data Processing

The database design will affect the quality of the data. A well designed database should be user friendly, and should incorporate filters, ranges and logical conditions to help detect inconsistencies and errors. All data should be entered twice, and any inconsistencies detected should be resolved by rechecking the original forms.

Once the data have been reviewed and corrected, it is a good idea to make a preliminary analysis by generating descriptive statistics for each variable, scattergrams of pairs of variables, tables of selected categorical variables, etc.

The data processing program that will transform the information in the form into the variables necessary to classify the patient can then be applied.

Data Analysis

The final analysis depends on the study objectives. For example, the Spanish study made the following analyses:

Analysis of the total sample

- *Descriptive analysis*: Patient characteristics, type of coronary disease at the time of the procedure, results of diagnostic tests, and classification in the list of indications. Proportion of incomplete charts and information needed to classify the patient in the list of indications.
- *Univariate analysis*: Association between appropriateness and different variables such as patient characteristics, type of coronary disease, characteristics of the centre, etc.
- *Multivariate analysis*: Association between appropriateness and different variables, adjusted using logistic regression or classification techniques.

Individual analysis for each participating centre

- *Descriptive analysis* for each centre, similar to that done for the total sample.
- *Comparative analysis* for each centre, showing individual results in comparison to those of the total sample.

Conclusions /Publications

The study conclusions will, of course, depend on the results of the analysis. Caution should be exercised when drawing conclusions about the whole population based on the results obtained in the study sample. Generalising the results requires a correct estimation of the sampling errors for each variable, keeping in mind the sample design. These calculations and their interpretation will require the help of a specialist in sampling techniques.

The results of the study should be made available to the scientific community in a timely fashion. The appropriateness criteria may be disseminated in different ways: through an internal report circulated to physicians, a medical society journal, or through a web page on the Internet (see Chapter 12). Researchers will also want to make their study results available to the larger scientific community through articles in international peer-reviewed journals.

It is important to let those who have participated in the project know its results. Depending on the type of agreement previously made with the investigators, each centre may want to receive tables of results specific to their own centre, perhaps comparing them with the global study results. Copies of publications produced as a result of the research project should also be sent to all participants.

CHAPTER 11. APPLYING NECESSITY CRITERIA TO MEASURE UNDERUSE

Introduction

Although studies of underuse of care are much less frequent than those examining overuse, there is reason to believe that the measurement of underuse will become increasingly important. The drive for efficiency in the health-care system is heightening pressure on both providers and payers to drastically reduce inappropriate care. In the overzealous drive to do so, it is possible that underuse of care will affect more and more people. The issue of how to measure underuse in a valid and reliable way will thus be of increasing concern.

Much of what was written in chapter 10 about planning and carrying out a study to measure overuse applies equally well to studies designed to measure underuse. Here, we focus on three issues specifically related to the measurement of underuse, namely, the criteria themselves, the difficulty of defining the target population, and the problems in obtaining funding for these types of studies.

Necessity Criteria

One problem in measuring underuse is related to the criteria themselves. Few studies have actually *developed* criteria to measure underuse, and even fewer have *applied* them to a real population. Arguably, the relative newness of this concept may cause some panellists to produce overly generous criteria of medical "necessity" and therefore produce an unexpectedly high rate of underuse. As Kahan et al. (1994a) have emphasised, there is a fundamental distinction between the medical appropriateness of a procedure and its necessity. Performing a procedure may be appropriate, i.e., its potential benefits outweigh its inherent risks, but another option might be equally appropriate, including, perhaps, watchful waiting. Necessity, on the other hand, implies that the health benefits outweigh the health risks to such an extent that the physician must offer the procedure to the patient (though the patient is obviously free to decline the procedure). The difficulty for experts to differentiate between *appropriate* and *necessary* may cause them to confuse the two concepts and to rate the necessity of procedures too high. It is important to carry out studies, including comparative follow-up of patients receiving or not receiving necessary care, in order to refine the concept and criteria of necessary care.

Defining the Target Population

An important difference between measuring overuse and underuse of a procedure is in the definition of the target population to be sampled. Finding cases involving underuse of the procedure presents a more complicated situation. In fact, to thoroughly identify *all* cases of underuse, one would ideally have to look everywhere *except* among that small group of patients who have received the procedure (see Figure 20). Most such cases will be found among patients who present symptoms related to the procedure in question, for example, most cases of underuse of gastrointestinal endoscopy will be found among patients who have consulted a physician for abdominal symptoms. Some cases of underuse, however, will also be found among patients who consulted a physician for some other reason, or among those whose condition was misdiagnosed. For example, a patient with chest pain due to gastro-esophageal reflux symptoms might be misdiagnosed as having coronary artery disease and subjected to inappropriate tests and treatment. Other cases may even be found in persons in the general population who have not consulted a physician at all.

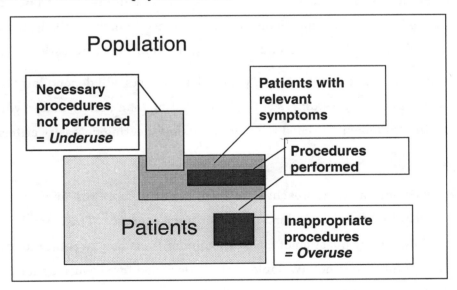

Figure 20. Underuse of Procedures. *Cases of underuse of a procedure will be found almost everywhere* **except** *among patients who have received the procedure.*

It is clearly impractical to survey the entire population of a country to identify all people who should have received a necessary medical or surgical procedure but did not, therefore innovative ways must be found to identify as many cases as possible, within the constraints of the available resources. The following examples show two approaches to targeting population groups who have a higher probability of meeting criteria for necessary care than those in the general population:

- In a study of the underuse of coronary revascularization (coronary artery bypass surgery and percutaneous transluminal coronary angioplasty), Kravitz et al. (1995) first identified a population of patients who had undergone coronary angiography. Among this group of patients they were then able to identify those who met necessity criteria for coronary revascularization.

- In a study on the underuse of upper gastrointestinal endoscopy (Froehlich et al., 1997), all patients evaluated at 20 primary care practices were first screened with a short questionnaire about the presence of gastrointestinal symptoms. For those who had such symptoms, the primary care physicians, who were blinded to the purpose of the study, completed a detailed questionnaire with information on patient history and physical examination. The questionnaire was designed to include all elements required to determine if endoscopy was appropriate or necessary.

The approach used to target such population sub-sets will depend largely on the resources and resourcefulness of the investigating team, and will also vary according to the elements needed to identify persons meeting necessity criteria.

Funding

Whatever innovative approaches are used, however, more resources will usually be required to study underuse than to study overuse. Thus, another problem related to the question of measuring underuse is how to obtain funding for the project. If funding is not available, a study designed to measure underuse will obviously never get off the ground. There is little motivation among funding sources to invest in measuring underuse, however, other than as a publicly funded academic research project. While *payers* are eager to detect and root out overuse, they are unlikely to be interested in seeking out areas where they will have to pay for the provision of additional care. *Physicians*, who might be interested in measuring underuse—from both an ethical and a financial perspective—infrequently fund research studies of this (or any other) nature. Given that underuse has been shown, in some studies, to be more prevalent in *underprivileged populations*, it is unreasonable to imagine that these populations will muster the political power to demand such studies.

On the other hand, if the increasing demand for greater equity in the health-care system prevails, this might help create the incentives to fund such studies, as would, of course, the extension of underuse to more influential segments of the population—a perspective that is not far-fetched.

Conclusions

If the concepts of appropriate and inappropriate care are fundamental to the creation of an efficient health-care delivery system, the notion of necessary care is vital to making that system equitable (Glassman et al., 1997). Evidence of underuse has been documented even in health systems characterised by the absence of global budgets, capitation, utilisation review or the pressure of requiring a second opinion. This leads us to believe it is perhaps even more widespread in other environments. It is therefore important that efforts be made to document and analyse underuse in different countries and for different procedures.

Health systems should function in such a way that inappropriate care is progressively reduced, while appropriate and especially necessary care are maintained or increased. The ability to determine and identify which care is overused and which is underused will be essential.

CHAPTER 12. APPLYING APPROPRIATENESS CRITERIA PROSPECTIVELY TO ASSIST IN DECISION-MAKING

The use of measures of appropriateness and necessity to retrospectively assess performance is relatively straightforward, at least conceptually. However, the potential benefits of such measures may be even greater if they can be used prospectively, as the basis for medical decision-making. This section describes some of the problems with retrospective performance audits and briefly presents three new approaches for using appropriateness criteria prospectively, so that physicians and, potentially, patients can have access to the recommendations of the expert panel. The first approach was developed at RAND and involves transforming the detailed appropriateness criteria into a set of user-friendly algorithms facilitating the use of the criteria. The second approach was developed by researchers at the Institute of Social and Preventive Medicine at the University of Lausanne and uses the Internet to make the panel recommendations available to interested users via a web page. In the third approach, designed by a group working in the Institute for Health Care Policy and Management at Erasmus University in Rotterdam, the recommendations are made available by means of a CD-ROM.

Problems with Retrospective Studies

Studies that have applied appropriateness criteria to real patients have yielded results such as those shown in Figure 21. This graph shows that a substantial proportion of care provided to patients over age 65 in the United States in the 1980s was inappropriate or, at best, its appropriateness was open to question.

With few exceptions, however, such studies have been carried out retrospectively, by reviewing medical records. There are several problems with such an approach. First, the medical record is not always precise enough to evaluate the appropriateness of care (e.g., Jeannot et al., 1999). Second, if the evaluator is aware of the outcome of care, he or she may be biased in assessing its appropriateness, with a positive outcome for an individual patient being more often associated with appropriate care (Caplan et al., 1991). Because many factors

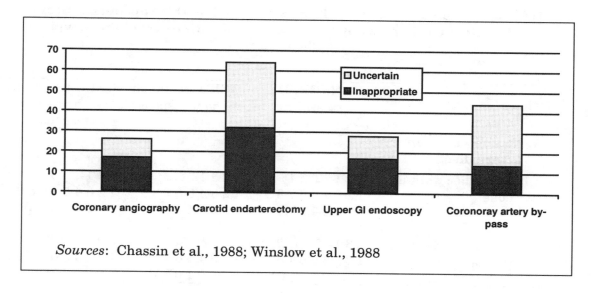

Figure 21. Examples of Proportion of Procedures Studied that are Inappropriate or Uncertain

besides the appropriateness and quality of care provided can affect patient outcome, such reasoning can be fallacious. Third, retrospective evaluation of care is of little use to the patient who has received inappropriate care and probably also to the physician who provided that care. Therefore, a key approach when moving from evaluating to improving the appropriateness of care is to provide both physicians and patients with access to the appropriateness criteria *before* the decision is made about care that is to be provided or received.

Obstacles to Prospective Use

Although the criteria developed by the RAM are attractive to practising physicians because of their clinical detail, at the same time this very characteristic hinders their actual use. The output from appropriateness panels is generally presented as hundreds and perhaps thousands of different clinical scenarios. Table 5 shows a small sample of the approximately 600 scenarios that were evaluated by the European panel on the appropriateness of gastrointestinal endoscopy. In each cell of this table the numbers above the 1-9 appropriateness scale indicate the votes of the 14 panel members. Below the appropriateness scale the median vote is indicated, followed by the absolute deviation from the median and the level of agreement among the panellists (A = agreement, D = disagreement).

Table 5. Sample Ratings from European Panel on the Appropriateness of Gastrointestinal Endoscopy for Selected Indications Involving Atypical Chest Pain

	No GERD treatment	GERD treatment without response	GERD treatment with positive response
A. No known coronary artery disease			
1. No cardiac work-up done	8 2 1 2 1 1 2 3 4 5 6 7 8 9 (1.0 1.36 A)	7 2 3 1 1 2 3 4 5 6 7 8 9 (2.0 1.14 A)	4 6 1 1 2 1 2 3 4 5 6 7 8 9 (2.0 1.36 A)
2. Cardiac work-up normal	2 3 1 3 3 2 1 2 3 4 5 6 7 8 9 (5.0 2.36 D)	2 5 3 4 1 2 3 4 5 6 7 8 9 (8.0 1.07 A)	3 2 3 1 3 2 1 2 3 4 5 6 7 8 9 (3.0 2.36 D)

Appropriateness scale: 1 = extremely inappropriate, 5 = uncertain, 9 = extremely appropriate.

It can readily be understood that a physician will find it quite impractical to wade through hundreds of such tables looking for the clinical scenario representing a particular patient before deciding whether it would be appropriate to request or perform a gastroscopy to elucidate the nature of the patient's symptoms.

An Algorithmic Approach

In an initial effort to improve the accessibility and use of appropriateness criteria, researchers at RAND converted standard appropriateness criteria for hysterectomy, developed in 1993, into a set of recommendations (Leape et al., 1997). An algorithm was developed in a multi-stage process that began with appropriateness ratings of 2,332 indications. Researchers turned these into guidelines presented in a flow chart format that was tested for user-friendliness. A national advisory panel then reviewed the guidelines, reduced the classification scheme to 102 unique indications, and turned the guidelines into clinical recommendations that emphasised the distinction between indications for which hysterectomy may sometimes be appropriate from those in which hysterectomy is clearly inappropriate except in unusual circumstances. Finally, the recommendations were reviewed for applicability and usefulness by a local panel of physicians in Southern California.

Figure 22 shows the algorithm for patients presenting with premenopausal abnormal uterine bleeding of unknown aetiology. By following the algorithm the patient can be classified as being a possible candidate or an inappropriate candidate for hysterectomy. Additionally, the physician can also clearly see what additional tests or treatments are recommended prior to considering hysterectomy for the patient. This is because hysterectomy may be considered an inappropriate treatment, not because the patient will not ultimately need the procedure, but because there may have been an inadequate evaluation (e.g., failure to obtain an endometrial sample prior to hysterectomy in a patient with abnormal uterine bleeding) or inadequate treatment (e.g., failure to try pain medications in a patient with pelvic pain) prior to referral for hysterectomy.

A WWW-Based Approach

Investigators at the Institute of Social and Preventive Medicine in collaboration with the Laboratory for Theoretical Computing at the Federal Institute of Technology, both at the University of Lausanne, have developed a web-based technology to make appropriateness criteria available to physicians and, eventually, to patients (Vader and Burnand, 1999). Two versions on line (as of June 2000) provide access to criteria from an expert panel convened in Switzerland in 1995 to examine the appropriateness of indications for low-back surgery (http://www.hospvd.ch/public/laminectomy/welc.htm) and to criteria from a European panel convened in 1999 to examine the appropriateness of gastrointestinal endoscopy (http://www.epage.ch).

Figure 23 shows the menu for the clinical scenarios for low-back surgery involving acute or sub-acute sciatica. By responding to six questions, the physician is immediately pointed to the panel results about the appropriateness of performing low-back surgery for patients with similar characteristics.

Figure 24 shows a view of the results page that would be obtained for an individual with the following presentation: sub-acute sciatica (lasting fewer than 6 weeks), with major muscular weakness and a herniated disk on radiological imaging. The patient has already been treated with one non-operative treatment regimen, and is severely disabled. The results indicate that for such a patient low-back surgery would be considered appropriate, with votes of the experts ranging from 5 to 9 on the nine-point scale. Elsewhere on the same web page, access is provided to summaries of articles from the medical literature concerning the efficacy, outcomes and complications of low-back surgery.

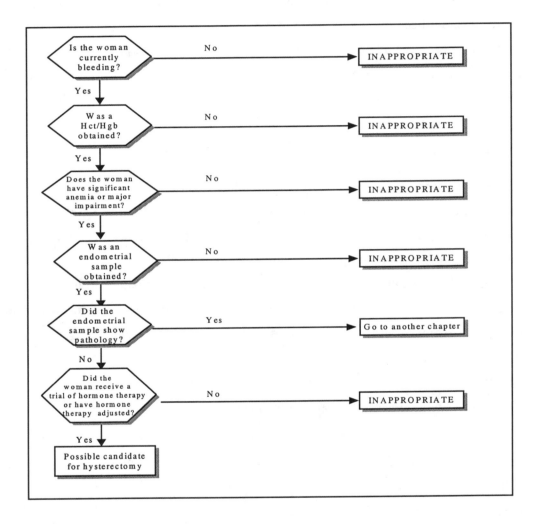

Source: Leape et al., 1997

Figure 22. Hysterectomy for Premenopausal Abnormal Uterine Bleeding of Unknown Aetiology

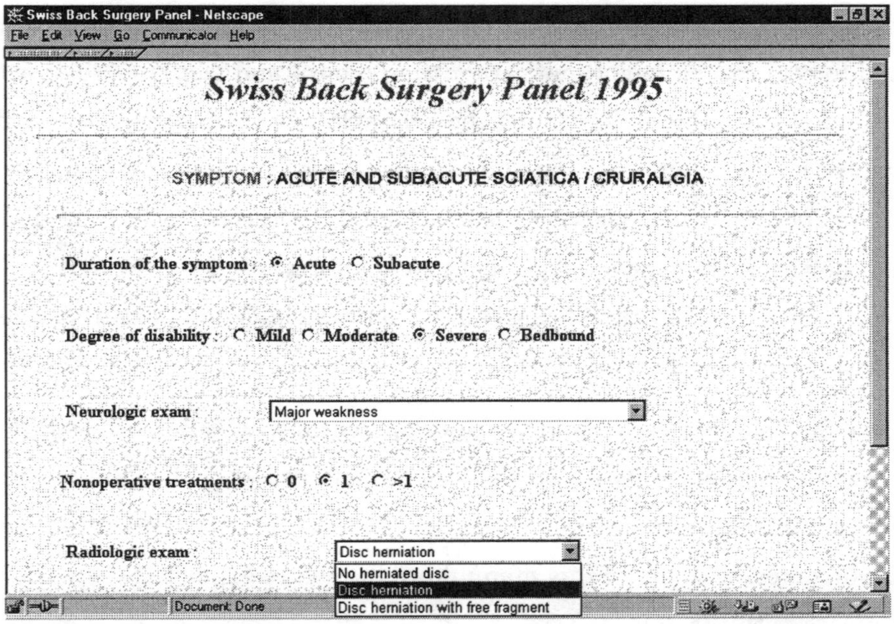

Figure 23. Sample page from WWW Instrument for Prospective Evaluation of the Appropriateness of Low-back Surgery

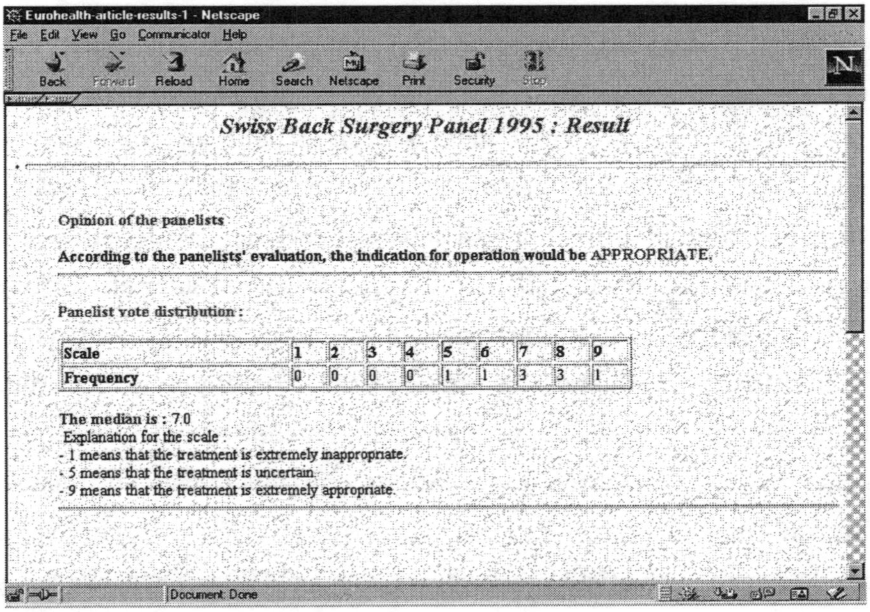

Figure 24. Partial View of Results Section of WWW Instrument Designed to Assist in the Evaluation of the Appropriateness of Low-back Surgery

The panel results concerning the appropriateness of an intervention are intended to be a recommendation, rather than a hard and fast rule, to assist patient and physician in determining the best strategy of care given the particular circumstances. It would be wrong and in some cases even harmful to base the decision to operate or not solely on the basis of such a recommendation. It is believed, however, that the availability of such information, via the WWW, for example, would provide valuable assistance to physicians and patients in deciding about the best course of care.

These instruments are still in the developmental stage and will need to be tested for their acceptability to physicians and patients, their feasibility of use, and their validity in terms of providing more appropriate care and optimising patient outcomes. Readers of this manual are invited to explore these websites and communicate with the developers.

A CD-ROM Approach

Given the often complex structure of the panel data and the large number of variables included, it is not easy to translate the results of appropriateness panels into comprehensive and convenient written recommendations. In order to handle this problem, the Institute for Health Care Policy and Management at Erasmus University, Rotterdam, has developed a software package that facilitates the use of the panel recommendations in daily clinical practice (Stoevelaar et al., 1999). The first application of this computer programme was based on the results of a BIOMED multinational panel on the appropriate treatment of benign prostatic hyperplasia. Figure 25 shows the user interface for the software package developed to make the panel recommendations available to users by means of a CD-ROM. On the left side, the patient's diagnostic characteristics are selected. The example shown in the figure describes a man aged 70 or over who has severe, non-specific symptoms which he considers unacceptable, and who has not been tried on alpha-blockers; he has had fewer than two urinary tract infections, his peak urinary flow rate is between 10 and 15 ml/s, his prostate volume is less than 30 ml, and his post-void residual urine volume is 150 ml or greater.

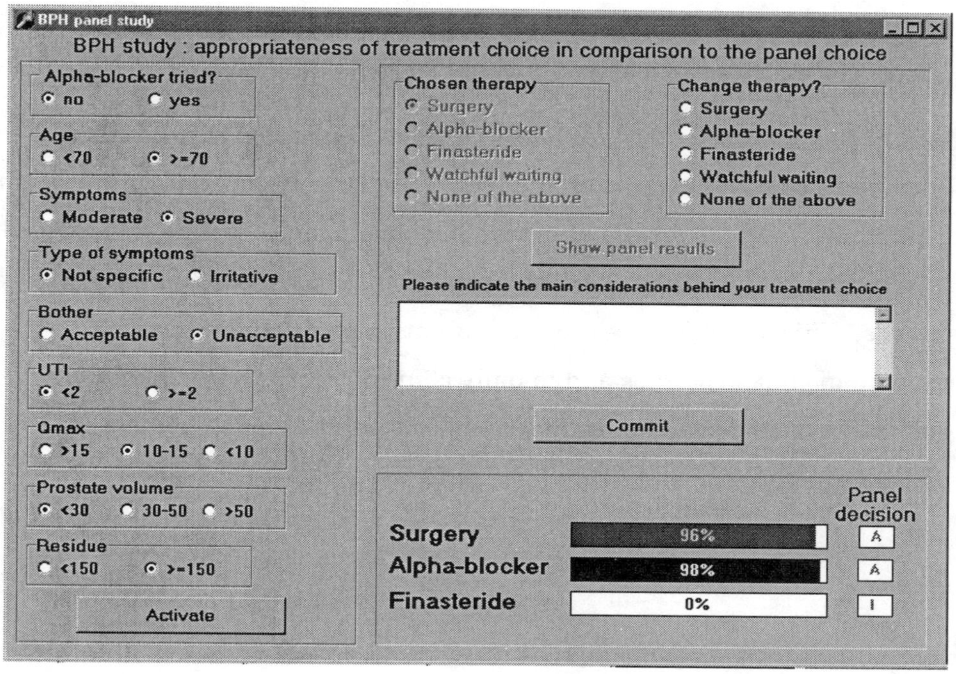

Figure 25. **User Interface for Software Designed to Compare Treatment Choice for Benign Prostatic Hyperplasia with Recommendations of a Dutch Expert Panel**

The program then asks the user to indicate the initial treatment choice by clicking on one of the treatments listed under "Chosen therapy" (in the example given, "Surgery" was chosen). Subsequently the panel recommendations are shown in two forms: 1) Text boxes (the squares below the column labelled "Panel decision" in the lower right-hand corner) indicate the actual ratings for the selected indication. In the example shown, the panel had rated both surgery and alpha-blocker treatment as appropriate (A), whereas finisteride treatment was inappropriate (I). 2) The gauges in the lower right-hand corner express the results of a logistic regression analysis over all indications. This analysis seeks to determine the underlying pattern of contributions made by the variables, uncontaminated by 'random noise' at the individual indication level. The percentages depicted in these gauges represent the probability that the panel would consider the treatments as being appropriate, each in comparison to the option of "no active treatment," if the RAM rating process were to be carried out again. Thus, in this example, the regression analysis shows that it is highly likely (96% for surgery and 98% for alpha-blocker treatment) that subsequent panels would again find these treatments to be appropriate, whereas there is virtually no likelihood that finasteride treatment would be rated appropriate.

After the panel recommendations are shown, the urologist is offered the opportunity to change his decision (under "Change therapy?") and to document the principal considerations for the alternate treatment choice in this patient. All data, including potential changes in treatment choice, are automatically stored in a database. This database enables the evaluation and validation of the programme in clinical studies and in daily clinical practice. It is planned to test the suitability of this programme in a number of studies involving different European countries.

CHAPTER 13. METHODOLOGICAL ISSUES

Reliability and Validity

The appropriateness method has been criticised on the grounds that the results obtained may well vary depending on the composition of the panel of experts selected, that is, the process may lack reliability. The most important study carried out to test the reproducibility of the method (Shekelle et al., 1998b) suggests that the method may be more reliable for some surgical procedures than for others. In this study, three separate panels were carried out for each of two procedures: coronary revascularization and hysterectomy. Panel members were selected from a list of experts nominated by the relevant speciality societies and assigned randomly to one of three parallel panels. Each panel independently rated the same set of clinical indications, for both appropriateness and necessity in the case of coronary revascularization, and for appropriateness only in the case of hysterectomy. In general, the authors found that for coronary revascularization they obtained good reliability for appropriateness and excellent reliability for necessity. However, the reliability with regard to hysterectomy was, although comparable to other methods for determining appropriateness, less than adequate. Based upon these findings, a likely conjecture—requiring further study—is that the RAM is most reliable (and therefore valid) when there is a solid scientific foundation of evidence from which the panel can extrapolate and when appropriateness is based upon relatively objective outcomes and processes.

What is clear from a number of studies is that clinical speciality has a strong influence on appropriateness ratings. In general, expert panels made up of same-discipline physicians rate more indications as appropriate than do panels composed of multiple specialities (Leape et al., 1992; Coulter et al., 1995). It has also been seen that, in multidisciplinary panels, those panel members who perform the procedure under study consistently have the highest mean ratings, followed by physicians in related specialities, while primary care providers have the lowest (Kahan et al., 1995; Fitch et al., 1999). These results support the recommendation that expert panels should include participation from a variety of relevant disciplines. They also further underline the fact that appropriateness criteria, by themselves, cannot be considered as a "gold standard" for practice decisions, but rather as a starting point for discussion of the relative risks and benefits of applying a procedure to a particular patient.

Another important methodological issue in the RAND/UCLA method is the extent to which the appropriateness and necessity criteria produced are valid, that is, whether they truly represent appropriate and necessary care for the clinical indication described (Fitch and Lázaro, 1999). One way to test the validity of the criteria is to determine if patients treated in accordance with the criteria have better outcomes than those who receive another (or no) treatment. In a study of underuse of coronary revascularization, the validity of the necessity criteria produced by a U.S. panel was examined by looking at the outcomes of patients undergoing coronary angiography who met necessity criteria for revascularization (Kravitz et al, 1995). It was found that adjusted mortality was lower among those who had received a necessary revascularization procedure than among those who had not. The study also found significantly fewer self-reported symptoms of angina among patients who had received a necessary revascularization.

Another study (Shekelle, 1998a; Chassin and Park, 1998) took advantage of a natural experiment to assess the predictive validity of appropriateness criteria for carotid endarterectomy. At the time of the first carotid endarterectomy appropriateness panel in 1984, only one randomised controlled trial (RCT) had been carried out, thus, very little scientific evidence was available to the panellists in making their ratings. Over the following 14 years, information about the efficacy of the procedure became available from six more RCTs. In comparing the expert panel appropriateness ratings with the results of the subsequent RCTs, the authors found that the trials confirmed the ratings for 44 indications in the list, which represented about 30% of the carotid endarterectomies performed on real patients, and refuted none of the ratings.

Resolving Inconsistencies

Another methodological issue that may need to be addressed when applying the RAM is concerned with the detection and correction of possible inconsistencies in the appropriateness ratings. It should not be surprising that, when panellists are asked to rate hundreds and perhaps thousands of clinical scenarios, occasional inconsistencies in the final appropriateness classification may occur. For example, if coronary revascularization is appropriate for a particular patient who has a negative stress test result, it does not seem logical to classify the procedure as inappropriate for the same patient with a positive stress test result. Likewise, if revascularization is appropriate for a patient on sub-optimal medical therapy it would be surprising to find a less than appropriate classification for a patient with the same combination of symptoms and disease characteristics who is on optimal medical therapy. Detecting these types of inconsistencies requires a combination of logic and clinical knowledge, as well as familiarity with the latest scientific evidence, since some seemingly logical inconsistencies may actually have a clinical explanation. Although two studies (Kravitz et al., 1997; McDonnell et al., 1996) have shown that inconsistencies are generally few in number, this is still a potential cause for concern.

Different methods have been applied in an attempt to resolve these kinds of inconsistencies. In the 1996 Spanish panel on the appropriateness of coronary revascularization procedures, it was decided to re-convene the panel to consider 90 potential inconsistencies (out of some 2000 indications). An analysis of the ratings for the inconsistent indications showed that they were generally borderline situations in which a small shift in ratings by one or two panellists would have changed the appropriateness classification. At the panel meeting, each type of inconsistency was discussed separately (for example, those pertaining to stress test results, medical therapy, ejection fraction and so on). The panellists unanimously agreed to change some of the appropriateness classifications, in almost all cases, from less appropriate to more appropriate, that is, from inappropriate to uncertain or from uncertain to appropriate.

In other cases, it may not be feasible to ask the panel members to meet again. The European endoscopy/colonoscopy panel, which included 14 experts from 9 countries, plans to resolve the approximately 20 inconsistencies detected (out of 600 indications) by correspondence with the panel members.

Another possible approach might be to phone the panellists, either individually or during a conference call, having previously asked that each person have the list of indications in front of them for the discussion. This method has been used in a U.S. appropriateness panel, but is only practical when there are a relatively small number of inconsistencies to be resolved.

Obsolescence

The problem of obsolescence arises from the fact that panellists rate appropriateness based on the scientific evidence available at the time of the panel meeting. Although the method has been shown to be a good "predictor" of developing evidence (Shekelle, et al., 1998a), any set of appropriateness criteria is at risk of obsolescence. Not only the appropriateness of indications, but the indications themselves may change over time, as both evidence and experience evolve. For example, new instruments or techniques may be developed which make it possible to perform procedures on patients who were previously not considered candidates because the risks were too high. New scientific knowledge is generated at such a rapid pace that what was once inappropriate may soon cease to be so, and the converse may also be true.

An important challenge to the RAM, therefore, is how to update the appropriateness criteria in "real time," as new evidence becomes available. One promising approach might be based on the use of Evidence Based Medicine techniques, combined with computers and the Internet, to assure that appropriateness criteria reflect the latest available scientific evidence.

Rigidity

Another important attribute of appropriateness criteria is that they should be flexible. However, as they are usually disseminated in paper format they most often exhibit the opposite attribute: rigidity. Thus, a physician may not be comfortable following the recommendations for a specific indication, for various reasons. For example, the local characteristics of a particular Cardiology or Cardiovascular Surgery Department may make it more reasonable to choose an option different from that recommended by the expert panel because the centre is highly atypical with regard to experience or equipment (recall that panellists are asked to base their ratings on an "average patient" presenting to an "average physician" practising in an "average health care setting"). Conversely, patients may prefer a different option than recommended by the criteria, for example, because of their perception of the risk involved, religious values or other considerations.

Resolving these limitations using a paper format is not practical. However, by using an interactive algorithm in the Internet, this limitation could be overcome.

The objective would be to make the criteria flexible, that is, adaptable to specific local situations. Appropriateness criteria should not limit physician freedom, but should impede arbitrary decisions. The difference between freedom and arbitrariness is that freedom permits decisions different from those recommended by the criteria, but requires that such decisions be justified. Arbitrariness means that the recommendations are not followed but no attempt is made to explain why. The idea is that physicians are free to choose a different (or no) alternative, so long as they explain the reason for their choice. The argument may be as simple as "In my hospital procedure X has not yet been sufficiently well developed, therefore it is better to apply procedure Y." To document the decision, the physician could simply write a short explanation in a text box. The physician's reason, once typed in, would go to a central web page where the exceptions to the recommendations would be analysed and possibly introduced as another option for users, depending on their frequency. Alternatively, the physician's reasoning may be incorrect and this could be directly addressed.

Dissemination

To date, most appropriateness criteria have been disseminated in paper format, either through internal publications or as articles in specialised medical journals (e.g., Lázaro et al., 1998). Neither of these formats is interactive. Furthermore, identifying where a particular patient fits in the indications matrix is difficult, time-consuming and requires familiarity with the structure of the list of indications. If the recommendations change in light of new evidence, it is difficult or impossible to re-circulate a new document with the revised criteria or have it published again in a medical journal. However, if the criteria were available in an interactive way on the Internet or by other electronic means, they could be disseminated quickly in a user-friendly fashion.

The best examples of how this type of approach has been implemented thus far are described in Chapter 12 ("A WWW-Based Approach" and "A CD-ROM Approach"). Another possibility would be to make the criteria available through the web page of the relevant medical society. For example, the appropriateness criteria produced by the Spanish expert panel on PTCA and CABG could be offered to the Spanish Society of Cardiology for inclusion in their web page. In 1998 this society reported receiving 1000 visits to their web page per week, a figure that is progressively rising. Such sites are being used by ever larger numbers of both physicians and patients, and they are likely to become increasingly important as the technology becomes more widespread and easier to use.

REFERENCES

Bernstein SJ, Hofer TP, Meijler AP, et al. Setting standards for effectiveness: a comparison of expert panels and decision analysis. *International Journal of Quality in Health Care* 1997; 9:255-263.

Bochud M, Burnand B, de Bosset V, et al. European Gastrointestinal Endoscopy: 1998 Literature Review. Lausanne, Institut universitaire de médecine sociale et préventive, 1998.

Broder MS, Kanouse DE, Mittman BS, et al. The appropriateness of recommendations of hysterectomy. *Obstetrics & Gynecology* 2000; 95: 199-205.

Brook RH. The RAND/UCLA appropriateness method. In: McCormick KA, Moore SR, Siegel RA (1994), Methodology Perspectives, AHCPR Pub. No. 95-0009, Rockville, MD: Public Health Service, U.S. Department of Health and Human Services, pp. 59-70.

Brook RH. Ensuring delivery of necessary care in the U.S. Statement before the U.S. Senate Committee on Health, Education, Labor and Pensions, 2 March 1999.

Brook RH, Chassin MR, Fink A, et al. A method for the detailed assessment of the appropriateness of medical technologies. *International Journal of Technology Assessment in Health Care.* 1986; 2(1): 53-63.

Caplan RA, Posner KL, Cheney FW. Effect of outcome on physician judgments of appropriateness of care. *JAMA* 1991; 265: 1957-1960.

Chalmers I. The Cochrane collaboration: preparing, maintaining, and disseminating systematic reviews of the effects of health care. *Annals of the New York Academy of Sciences* 1993; 703: 156-163.

Chassin MR, Kosecoff J, Park RE, et al. Does inappropriate use explain geographic variations in the use of health care services? A study of three procedures. *JAMA* 1987; 258 (18): 2533-2537.

Coulter I, Adams A, Shekelle PG. Impact of varying panel membership on ratings of appropriateness in consensus panels: a comparison of a multi- and single disciplinary panel. *Health Services Research* 1995; 30: 577-591.

Fink A, Kosecoff J, Chassin M, et al. Consensus methods: characteristics and guidelines for use. *American Journal of Public Health* 1984; 74:979-983.

Fitch K, Lázaro P. Using appropriateness criteria to improve health care. *Eurohealth* 1999; 5 (3): 19-21.

Fitch K, Lázaro P, Martin Y, Bernstein S. Physician recommendations for coronary revascularization: Variations by clinical specialty. *European Journal of Public Health* 1999; 8: 517-524.

Froehlich P, Pache I, Burnand B, et al. Underutilisation of upper gastrointestinal endoscopy. *Gastroenterology* 1997; 112: 690-697.

Glassman PA, Model KE, Kahan JP et al. The illusion of deterministic rules in decisions invoking medical necessity and cost-effectiveness. *Annals of Internal Medicine* 1997; 126: 152-156.

Goodman C. Literature searching and evidence interpretation for assessing health care practices. Stockholm: The Swedish Council on Technology Assessment in Health Care, 1993.

Jeannot JG, Vader JP, Porchet F, et al. Can the decision to operate be judged retrospectively? A study of medical records. *European Journal of Surgery* 1999; 165:516-521.

Johansson SR, Brorsson B, Bernstein SJ. Coronary artery bypass graft and percutaneous transluminal coronary aniolasty: A literature review and ratings of appropriateness and necessity. The Swedish Council on Technology Assessment, SBU Report No. 120E, May 1994.

Kahan JP, Bernstein SJ, Leape LL, et al. Measuring the necessity of medical procedures. *Medical Care* 1994; 32: 357-365. (a)

Kahan, JP, Morton SC, Farris HH, et al. Panel processes for revising relative values of physician work: A pilot study. *Medical Care* 1994; 32: 1069-1085. (b)

Kahan JP, Park RE, Leape LL, et al. Variations by specialty in physician ratings of the appropriateness and necessity of indications for procedures. *Medical Care* 1995; 34 (6): 512-523

Kahan JP, Loo M van het. Defining appropriate health care. *Eurohealth* 1999; 5 (3): 16-18.

Kanouse DE, Brook RH, Winkler JD, et al. Changing medical practice through technology assessment: an evaluation of the NIH Consensus Development Program. RAND Report No. R-3452-NIH/RC, 1989.

Kosecoff J, Fink A, Brook RH, et al. The appropriateness of using a medical procedure. Is information in the medical record valid? *Medical Care* 1987; 25: 196-201.

Kravitz RL, Laouri M, Kahan JP, et al. Validity of criteria used for detecting underuse of coronary revascularization. *JAMA*. 1995; 274: 632-638.

Kravitz RL, Park RE, Kahan JP. Measuring the clinical consistency of panelists' appropriateness ratings: The case of coronary artery bypass surgery. *Health Policy* 1997; 42: 135-143.

Kuntz KM, Tsevat J, Weinstein MC, et al. Expert panel vs decision-analysis recommendations for postdischarge coronary angiography after myocardial infarction. *JAMA* 1999; 282: 2246-2251.

Lázaro P, Fitch K, Martín Y. Estándares para el uso apropiado de la angioplastia coronaria transluminal percutánea y cirugía aorto-coronaria (Criteria for the appropriate use of percutaneous transluminal coronary angioplasty and coronary artery bypass graft surgery). *Revista Española de Cardiología* 1998; 51: 689-715

Leape LL, Hilborne LE, Kahan JP, et al. Coronary artery bypass graft: A literature review and ratings of appropriateness and necessity. Santa Monica: RAND Corporation, Publication No. JRA-02, 1991.

Leape LL, Park RE, Kahan JP, et al. Group judgments of appropriateness: the effect of panel composition. *Quality Assurance in Health Care* 1992; 4: 151-159.

Leape LL, Bernstein SJ, Bohon CJ, et al. Hysterectomy: Clinical Recommendations and Indications for Use. RAND, Santa Monica, MR-592/1, 1997.

Linstone, H.A., M. Turoff. The Delphi method: Techniques and applications. Reading Massachusetts: Addison-Wesley. 1975.

Loo M van het, Kahan JP. The RAND Appropriateness Method: An Annotated Bibliography through June 1999. Leiden: RAND Europe. Report No. RE/99.010. June 1999.

McDonnell J, Meijler A, Kahan JP, et al. Panelist consistency in the assessment of medical appropriateness. *Health Policy* 1996; *37:* 139-152.

Park RE, Fink A, Brook RH, et al. Physician ratings of appropriate indications for six medical and surgical procedures. *American Journal of Public Health.* 1986; 76 (7): 766-772

Rowe MK, Kanouse DE, Mittman BS, et al. Quality of life among women undergoing hysterectomies. *Obstetrics & Gynecology* 1999; 93(6): 915-921.

Shekelle PG, Chassin MR, Park RE. Assessing the predictive validity of the RAND/UCLA appropriateness method criteria for performing carotid endarterectomy. *International Journal of Technology Assessment in Health Care* 1998a; 14: 707-727.

Shekelle PG, Kahan JP, Bernstein SJ, et al. The reproducibility of a method to identify the overuse and underuse of medical procedures. *New England Journal of Medicine* 1998b; 338: 1888-1895.

Stoevelaar HJ, McDonnell J, Bosch JLH, et al. Appropriate treatment of benign prostatic hyperplasia: A European panel study. Rotterdam: Institute for Health Care Policy and Management, Erasmus University, 1999.

Vader JP, Burnand B. Prospective assessment of the appropriateness of health care. *Eurohealth* 1999; 5 (3): 21-23.

Winslow CM, Kosecoff J, Chassin MR, et al. The appropriateness of performing coronary artery bypass surgery. *JAMA* 1988; 260: 505-509.

ANNEX I. Members of the European Union BIOMED Concerted Action on "A Method to Integrate Scientific and Clinical Knowledge to Achieve the Appropriate Utilisation of Major Medical and Surgical Procedures"

Institution	Persons to Contact
RAND EUROPE Newtonweg 1 2333 CP Leiden, The Netherlands tel: 31-71-524.51.51 fax: 31-71-524.51.91	James P. **Kahan** (kahan@rand.org) Mirjam **van het Loo** (m.vanhetloo@randeurope.org) Ineke **van Beusekom** (i.vanBeusekom@randeurope.org)
CARLOS III HEALTH INSTITUTE Unidad de Investigación en Servicios de Salud Instituto de Salud Carlos III Calle Sinesio Delgado, 6 28029 Madrid, Spain tel: 34-91-387.78.03 fax: 34-91-387.78.96	Pablo **Lázaro** (plazaro@isciii.es) Kathy **Fitch** (kfitch@isciii.es) María Dolores **Aguilar** (daguilar@isciii.es)
ERASMUS UNIVERSITY Erasmus Universiteit Rotterdam Institut voor Beleid en Management van de Gezondheidszorg (iBMG) 3000 DR Rotterdam, The Netherlands tel: 31-10-408.85.62 fax: 31-10-408.90.92	Herman **Stoevelaar** (stoevelaar@bmg.eur.nl) Joseph **McDonnell** (mcdonnell@bmg.eur.nl)
GALDAKAO HOSPITAL Unidad de Investigación Hospital de Galdakao Barrio Labeaga s/n 48960 Galdakao, Vizcaya, Spain tel: 34-94-457.13.27 fax: 34-94-456.62.68	José María **Quintana** (jmquinta@hgda.osakidetza.net)
INSTITUTE OF PREVENTIVE AND SOCIAL MEDICINE - LAUSANNE Institut Universitaire de Médecine Sociale et Préventive (IUMSP) 17, Rue de Bugnon 1005 Lausanne, Switzerland tel: 41-21-314.72.55 fax: 41-21-314.73.73	Bernard.**Burnand** (Bernard.Burnand@inst.hospvd.ch) John Paul **Vader** (John-Paul.Vader@inst.hospvd.ch) Vincent **Wietlisbach** (Vincent.Wietlisbach@inst.hospvd.ch) Valerie **Pittet** (Valerie.Pittet@inst.hospvd.ch)
INSTITUTE FOR SOCIAL AND PREVENTIVE MEDICINE - ZURICH Institut für Sozial- und Präventivmedizin Sumatrastrasse 30 CH 8006 Zürich, Switzerland tel: 41-1-634.85.90 fax: 41-1-634.85.98	Julian **Schilling** (juli@ifspm.unizh.ch) Karin **Faisst** (caro@ifspm.unizh.ch)

LEUVEN SCHOOL OF PUBLIC HEALTH
Katholieke Universiteit Leuven
Postbus 214
3000 Leuven, Belgium
tel: 32-16-33.69.78
fax: 32-16-33.69.70

Mia **Defever** (Mia.Defever@med.kuleuven.ac.be)
Katrien **Kesteloot**
(katrien.kesteloot@uz.kuleuven.ac.be)

MARIO NEGRI INSTITUTE
Via Eritrea 62
20157 Milan, Italy
tel: 39-02-39.01.45.14
fax: 39-02-33.20.02.31

Roberto **Grilli** (currently at Agenzia per i Servizi
Sanitari Regionali, Rome, Italy)
Alessandro **Liberati (currently at University of
Modena)**

**SWEDISH COUNCIL ON TECHNOLOGY
ASSESSMENT IN HEALTH CARE (SBU)**
Box 16158
10327 Stockholm, Sweden
tel: 46-8-412.32.00
fax: 46-8-412.32.60

Bengt **Brorsson** (brorsson@sbu.se)

UNIVERSITY HOSPITAL CENTER
Service Epidémiologie
Economie de la Santé et Prévention
Hotel-Dieu, Centre Hospitalier Universitaire
B.P. 69
63003 Clermont-Ferrand Cedex 1, France
tel: 33-4-73-31.61.81
fax: 33-4-73-31.61.01

Laurent **Gerbaud** (lgerbaud@chu-clermontferrand.fr)
Juliette **Deboursse**
Gerard **Manhès**

**UNIVERSITY OF MICHIGAN MEDICAL
CENTER**
Department of Internal Medicine
Division of General Medicine
The University of Michigan, Medical Center
Ann Arbor, Michigan 48109-0376 (USA)
tel: 1-734-647-96.88
fax: 1-734-936.89.44

Steven J. **Bernstein** (sbernste@umich.edu)

VALME UNIVERSITY HOSPITAL
Medicina Interna
Hospital Universitario de Valme
Ctra de Cádiz, s/n
41014 Sevilla, Spain
tel: 34-95-459.62.70
fax: 34-95-469.37.57

Ignacio **Marín** (miniml@valme.sas.cica.es)
Juan Ramón **Lacalle Remigio** (lacalle@cica.es)

ANNEX II. List of Acronyms

AI	Asymmetry Index
BPH	Benign Prostatic Hyperplasia
CABG	Coronary Artery Bypass Graft surgery
CFI	Correction Factor for Asymmetry
ECACIS	Estudio de la Calidad de la Asistencia a la Cardiopatía Isquémica en Sevilla (Study of the Quality of Care for Cardiac Ischemia in Sevilla)
IPR	Interpercentile Range
IPRAS	Interpercentile Range Adjusted for Symmetry
LVEF	Left Ventricular Ejection Fraction
MESH	Medical Subject Heading
NGT	Nominal Group Technique
NIH	National Institutes of Health
PLAD	Proximal Left Anterior Descending (coronary vessel)
PTCA	Percutaneous Transluminal Coronary Angioplasty
RCT	Randomised Controlled Trial
RAM	RAND/UCLA Appropriateness Method
SCEDAN	Scenario Developer and Analyser
UCLA	University of California at Los Angeles
WWW	World Wide Web